Ripin Garewal
Jessica Garewal
Natasha Hayer

Clefts of Lip and Palate

A step by step contemporary guide of Diagnosis &
Treatment Planning

JustFiction Edition

Imprint

Any brand names and product names mentioned in this book are subject to trademark, brand or patent protection and are trademarks or registered trademarks of their respective holders. The use of brand names, product names, common names, trade names, product descriptions etc. even without a particular marking in this work is in no way to be construed to mean that such names may be regarded as unrestricted in respect of trademark and brand protection legislation and could thus be used by anyone.

Cover image: www.ingimage.com

Publisher:
JustFiction! Edition
is a trademark of
International Book Market Service Ltd., member of OmniScriptum Publishing Group
17 Meldrum Street, Beau Bassin 71504, Mauritius

Printed at: see last page
ISBN: 978-613-9-42455-9

Chapter-1

INTRODUCTION

Cleft lip and palate are one among the most common congenital anomalies, affecting the population. These defects pose problems right from the time the child is born.

Defects in feeding, speech, hearing, and personality and as for the dental aspect, malocclusions and dental anomalies are common in cleft lip and cleft palate patients. These defects have been taken into consideration and advanced research has been undertaken pertaining to the causative factors, and its role in development of clefts.

Today medical approach towards the cleft lip and palate has advanced to such an extend that could cure all defects associated with cleft lip and palate. The multidisciplinary approach has been undertaken as a gold standard to treat these defects, right from the birth. Treatment provided in this approach connects different faculties in order to attain definite results.

Parental attitudes towards children with developmental anomalies like cleft lip and palate need to be altered to a vast extent. These children no more have to be looked down in society due to the drastic transformation given to them by our modern advanced medical technology. Their life can be carried out as normal individuals.

In this review, an attempt has been made to review cleft lip and palate and modern trends in its management.

Chapter-2

HISTORICAL PERSPECTIVE

Facial Appearance

Man has been interested in the severe malformations of the cranio facial complex since time immemoral. Among jade carvings found in Central America, dating back to the first century AD, are several depicting clefts of the lip and palate.

Alberto Carrion Vergarra, a plastic surgeon who operated on many cleft lip patients that went down to Lima from the Andes, forwarded pictures of ceramic sculptures of clefts from the Museo Arqueologico of Lima dating from A.D. 200 to 400.

One specimen is a small red-brown and white figure with a central lip and nose deformity which appears to be a median cleft but could represent the ravages of leishmaniasis or punishment for adultery by mutilation.

Another is a black stirrup spout vessel, portraying with remarkable accuracy a bilateral cleft lip with a small prolabium.

The third is also a red-brown and white stirrup spout vase depicting perfectly the unilateral lip cleft with exposure of the distorted maxilla and a malpositioned tooth, a philtrum dimple and the typical nasal deformity[118].

In those days the abnormal facial appearance often associated with above – average intelligence, led to these unusual people being appointed leaders of their tribe or even tribal gods.

Xipi-Totec, the pre-Columbian Goddess of Fertility is represented as a human female with bilateral cleft lip. In the present age, such is the social and commercial significance of a pleasing facial appearance that those who fall below the norm for the species are often objects of humiliation and discrimination.

In some places many congenital deformities, including cleft lip and palate, were considered to be evidence of evil spirit in the afflicted child. These children were often removed from the tribe or cultural unit and left to die in the surrounding wilderness.

Treatment History

Surgeons through the ages have attempted to correct the abnormal anatomic arrangement of the cleft lip and palatal tissues and achieve a "normal" appearance.

Boo-Chai (1966) reported a case of successful closure of a cleft lip in approximately 390 A.D. in China, although the surgeon's name is not mentioned. In Europe many surgical techniques were used for the treatment of wounds during the early Christian era. Hot cautery was a special feature of Arabian surgery, whereas Greek and Roman surgeons favoured the scalpel.

Yperman (1295 – 1351) was a Flemish surgeon who appears to have written the first fully documented description of cleft lip and its surgical repair. He closed the freshened borders of the cleft lip with a triangular needle armed with a twisted wax suture, a common method of suture at the time.

Tagliacozzi (1597) described a lip closure that employed mattress sutures passed through all layers of the lip tissue. This was a departure from the prevailing technique of needle closure and figure-of-eight suture material reinforcement. Thus, in the sixteenth century, closure of cleft lip to improve appearance was widely practiced, and the need for closure of the cleft palate to improve speech was appreciated in more limited surgical circles.

Treatment of the protruding premaxilla using a head bandage to achieve external compression of the premaxillary segment, thereby reducing it to a more favourable position for lip closure, was introduced by Desault and Bichat[40] (1798). Over the years, various combinations of intraoral and extraoral devices were developed in order to reduce the protruding premaxillary segment and also to maintain the lateral arch segments in adequate anatomic relationship with the lower jaw.

At the present time, there is renewed interest in orthodontic (pin) appliances inserted into infants' mouths to recess the protruding premaxilla and expand the collapsed maxillary segments[69].

It has been postulated that the first obturation of a cleft palate was by Demosthenes (384-323 B.C.). Bien suggested that the great Greek orator visited the seashore to search for appropriately sized pebbles adequate to fill his palatal defect and thereby improve his speech.

More current medical literature credits Hollerius, Petronius, and Pare with descriptions of prostheses for obturation of palatal defects in the 16th century. Works by Snell, Stearn, Kingsley, and Suerson in the 19th century describe current prosthetic designs (Aramany,[7] 1971).

The origins of the present techniques for successful closure of the secondary cleft palate are found in the early work of Graefe and Roux, who in 1817 and 1819, respectively, closed the cleft of the soft palate with interrupted twine sutures. In Roux's patient, a dramatic change of voice was immediately noted and described.

The techniques of treatment for cleft lip and palate, therapy for ancillary problems such as dentoalveolar arch deformities, nasal abnormalities, maxillary hypoplasia, and speech difficulties have progressed to a point at which, in modern times, teams of specialists have been formed to manage the total problem, which has grown too complicated for one or two disciplines alone.

This concept of the multidisciplinary team for treatment and evaluation is especially important in the case of the more complex craniofacial anomalies (McCarthy, 1976, Munro,[69] 1981).

Chapter-3

INCIDENCE AND PREVALENCE

Epidemiologists make a careful distinction between the terms incidence and prevalence: "incidence" – denotes the number of new cases entering a population in a specified time period and "prevalence" - denotes the number of existing cases in the population at some time (Hook, 1988).

As we review the information on frequency of occurrence of cleft lip and palate, there are three points to keep in mind.

1. The accuracy of any set of numbers on the frequency of occurrence of clefts in a given population depends on how thoroughly each individual was examined. Unfortunately, a large number of studies have relied on information recorded on birth certificates and all congenital malformations are notoriously underreported on birth records.

2. At least one minor or one major additional anomaly accompanies more than half of all clefts. If the presence of additional anomalies is not recognized the CL/CP will be erroneously recorded as an isolated defect, a misktake that leads to errors in epidemiologic data and, more important, to errors in determining causation (on a population level) and in planning appropriate treatment for the patient.

3. As many submucous clefts remain undetected, estimates of the frequency of clefts in any given population are artificially low.

i) **Table 3.1- Incidence of clefts in the world**

Date	Source	Location	Incidece	Ratio to Normal Births
1. 4000-2000 B.C.	mummies	Egypt	1:1,000	1:1,000
2. A.D. 1864	Frobelius	Russia	118:180,000	1:1,525
3. 1908	Rischbieth	London	39:67,945	1:1,742
4. 1924	Davis	Baltimore	24:28,085	1:1,170
5. 1929	Peron	Paris	106:100,889	1:952
6. 1931	Schroder	Minister, Germany	28:34,000	1:1,214
7. 1931	Gunther	Leipzig. Germany	102:102,834	1:1,008
8. 1933	Sanders	Leiden, Holland	16:15,270	1:954
9. 1934	Grothkopf	Hamburg, Germany	74:47,200	1:950
10. 1934	Faltin	Finland		1:950
11. 1934	Sanvenero-Roselli	Italy		1:1,000
12. 1939	Edberg	Goreberg,		

5

			Sweden	28:27,00	1:964
13. 1939	Fogh-Andersen		Copenhagen	193:128,306	1:665
14. 1940	Conway	New York	32:22,513		1:704
15. 1940	Henderson		Hawaii	35:18,024	1:515
16. 1942	Grace		Pennsylvania	250:202,501	1:810
17. 1944	Mucller		Wisconsin	736:567,504	1:771
18. 1946	Hanhart		Switzerland		1:1,250
19. 1947	Phair		Wisconsin		1:770
20. 1949	Oldfield	England			1:600
21. 1949	Hixon		Ontario	695:655,332	1:943
22. 1950	Ivy		Pennsylvania	766:583,690	1:762
23. 1953	MacMohan		Birmingham	285:218,693	1:767
24. 1953	Wallace	New York			1:1,202
25. 1954	Douglas		Tennessee		1:1,694
26. 1955	Lending		New York		1:1,342
27. 1955	Lutz		California	70:72,107	1:1,030
28. 1955	Lorenz		California		1:851
29. 1958	Kung and Chu		China		1:1,000
30. 1958	Pleydell	Northampronshire, England			1:637
31. 1960	Sesgin and stark	New York	21:27,087		1:1,290
32. 1960	Rank and Thompson		Tasmania	160:96,510	1:603
33. 1960	Broadbent		Urah	89:59,000	1:663
34. 1961	Tretsven		Montana	229:123,114	1:538
35. 1961	Simikiss and Lowe		Africa	3:2,068	1:689
36. 1963	Robinson		Trinidad		1:857
37. 1964	Conway		New York	1,457:1,823,244	1:1,251
38. 1965	Longenecker		New Orleans	154:199,109	1:1,293
39. 1966	Niswander		Phoenix	50:25,340	1:507
40. 1969	Gopra		Nigeria		1:1,055
41. 1972	Carlisle		Phoenix	32:16,495	1:515
42. 1977	Lowry and Timble		Columbia	096:1000	
43. 1987	Chung		Hawaii	1:1000	
44. 1989	Margaret E.Cooper		Shangai	1.2:1000	
45. 1998	Croen		California	0.96:1000	
46. 1998	Croen		African – American	0.5:1000	
47. 1997	Christensen		Europe and North American	1:1000	
48. 2000	Sivaraju.S[136]		India	1:781.	

Frequency data by type of cleft

Fogh – Andersen[48] (1942) noted a distribution according to type of cleft of 25 percent cleft lip alone, 50 percent CL / CP, and 25 percent isolated CP among Danish cases. Ingalls, Taube, and Klinberg[64] (1964) reported a respective frequency of 16, 30, and 54 percent; Fraser and Calnan[52] (1961) reported 21, 46, and 33 percent, respectively.

Unilateral left–sided clefting, unilateral right–sided clefting and bilateral clefting occur in a 6:3:1 relationship (Wilson,[163] 1972). As noted by Fogh–Andersen and confirmed by other studies, there is a left sided preponderance of cleft lip, in addition, there is a male excess in CL / CP and a female excess in isolated CP. Cleft palate is more often associated with bilateral (86%) than with unilateral (68%) clefts of the lip and this finding is consistent with the concept that cleft palate is seen in the more severe type of lip deformities.

Racial Influences

It has long been known that the frequency of clefts varies significantly among racial groups but obviously the differences become less distinct as people from different racial backgrounds intermarry. Historically, epidemiologists have reported a higher frequency of CL/CPamong Asian or Mongolian people than among Caucasians, and the lowest frequency in Blacks.

The mean incidence of CL / CP in Caucasians is approximately one per 1000 population (Fraser[51], 1970). A higher frequency of CL / CP among Japanese infants was reported as approximately 2.1 per 1000; the incidence rate for CP was 0.00055 (Neel,[105] 1958). The data of Fujino, Tanaka, and Sanui[53] (1963) also support the findings of an increased frequency among Orientals.

Blacks in the United States have been extensively studied, and it was noted that Blacks are at considerably lower risk of CL / CP than are Caucasians. In a large collaborative survey of births in several university hospitals, the frequency of CL / CP per 1000 births was 1.34 for Whites and 0.41 for Blacks.

The differences in these three large groups are generally reported to be on the order of 2 to 1 to 0.5 (twice as many clefts in Asians as Caucasians, twice as many clefts in Caucasians as Blacks).

The racial background of American Indians is Mongolian, and the occurence of cleft lip with or without cleft palate is much higher than in Caucasians, with some variation according to the particular group under study. Vanderas[59] (1987) reviewed more than 60 studies on this topic and concluded that the highest rates for CL/CP occurred in North American Indians (as high as 3.74/1000, or 1 in 267), followed by the Japanese (0.82 to 3.36 per 1000, or 1 in 1219 to 1 in 297), the Chinese (1.45 to 4.04 per 1000, or 1 in 689 to 1 in 247), Caucasians (1 in 1000 to 1 in 372), and Blacks (0.18 to 1.67 per 1000, or 1 in 5555 to 1 in 598). The frequency of cleft lip with or without palate is also higher in Mexicans (De Voss,[39] 1952; Lutz and Moore,[84] 1955).

By contrast, the prevalence of clefts of the secondary palate is approximately the same among Caucasians, African – Americans, American – Indians and Asians.

Sex Ratio

In Whites, there is an excess of males with CL / CP, the proportion ranging from 60 to 80 percent (Drillien, Ingram, and Walkinson,[43] 1966). Fogh – Andersen (1942) noted that male preponderance is more marked in the more severe or complete CL / CP defects and in bilateral rather than unilateral clefts. Male excess in CL / CP is less pronounced among the Japanese (Fujino, Tanaka, and sanui[53], 1963).

Female excess has been reported in isolated CP (Fogh – Andersen[49] 1942, Fraser and Calnan[52] 1961). In addition, those clefts extending more anteriorly toward the incisive foramen are far more frequent in females.

Parental Age

There is some evidence that the risk of producing an affected child is decreased in younger parents and increased in older parents (Woolf [169]1963). Fraser and Calnan (1961) considered that the most important factor was elevated parental and not maternal age.

A significant positive relationship between parental age and isolated CP could not be demonstrated in a study of Caucasians (Woolf, Woolf and Broadbent,[168] 1963).

Reasons for increase in cleft incidence:

1. Simple improvement in clinical detection of cleft.

2. Steadily improving operative results:
   In Denmark, as in other parts of the world, an ever increasing number of men and women who were born with clefts go through successful habilitation (surgery, orthodontics, prosthodontics, speech – language services, psychosocial services, etc.) So that they become normal members of their social community, and as such, find partners and reproduce.

3. Falling perinatal mortality.

4. Decreased operative mortality
   Peron quoted a 13% mortality rate in the first 10 days of life, and Fogh – Andersen quoted a similar figure. In 1954 Ivy[65] reported that 10% died within the first year of life – nearly all had multiple congenital anomalies. In 1962 Lewin reported that of the 5000 infants with clefts born in Russia in one year, one – third died. Fogh – Andersen reported a reduction to 0.4% mortality (3 deaths in 900).

5. Attendant increase in fertility:

Molsted Pedersen (1964) reported a 1:170 (5 in 853) incidence of clefts in children born of diabetic mothers. Many who not so long ago would have died of grave illnesses like diabetes now have children.

6. Importance of Intermarriage:

Consanguinous marriages may account for rising incidence of cleft lift and palate in small countries such as Denmark, Finland, Greenland and Tasmania. Small communities like American Indians where marriage outside the tribe is frowned upon may account for the high incidence.

The Influence of Genetics

Grabb, Rosenstein, and Bzoch[118] (1971) published a book on cleft lip and palate. In that book, Fraser outlined the chances of parents having children with clefts, assuming that known genetic and chromosomal syndromes had been excluded. Noting the frequency of the defect in the general population to be 0.1% for CL with or without CP and 0.04% for CP, he correlated various situations with estimated percentages.

If both parents are unaffected and they have an affected child, the probability that their next baby will have the same condition if,

they have no affected relatives : 4% in CL with or without CP, 2% in CP

they have an affected relative : 4% in CL with or without CP, 7% in CP

they are related to each other :
Same as general population the affected child has another malformation
: 2% in CL with or without CP, 2% in CP.

If unaffected parents have two affected children, the probabilty that their next baby will have the same condition is 9% in CL with or without CP and 1% in CP.

If one parent is affected and they have no affected children, the probability of the next baby being affected is 4% in CL with or without CP and 6% in CP.

If one parent is affected and they have an affected child, the probability of the next baby being affected is 17% in CL with or without CP and 15% in CP.

If both parents are affected, Fraser estimated, assuming a heritability of 80%, the risk for the offspring would be about 60%. Their having one or two affected children increases the risk only slightly above this, presumably because the two affected parents contribute about all the "susceptibility" genes there are.

Other malformations:

It is puzzling that when there is another major malformation, which is not part of a genetic syndrome, the risk becomes smaller for recurrence of the cleft anomaly.

The degree of cleft

According to Carter, the more severe the patient's cleft, the higher the recurrence risk with 2.5% for unilateral cleft lip to 5 to 7% for bilateral cleft lip and palate.

A feminist trend

Both Carter and Woolf concur that the rate of recurrence is a little higher for females than males.

Chapter-4

EMBRYOLOGY OF CLEFT LIP AND PALATE

The primary palate forms the initial separation between the developing oral and nasal cavities. It eventually gives rise to much of the upper lip, the associated dentoalveolar ridge, and that portion of the hard palate infront of the incisive foramen. It appears that almost all cases of human cleft lip, with or without associated cleft palate are caused by failure of the medial nasal prominence (MNP) to make contact with lateral nasal prominence (LNP) and maxillary process.

The secondary palate completes the separation between the oral and nasal cavities by forming most of the hard palate and all of the soft palate. Almost all palatal clefts appear to result from the failure of the palatal shelves to make contact with each other.

Normal Palatal Closure

During the 8th week of intra uterine life a remarkable transformation in position of the lateral shelves takes place, when they alter from vertical to horizontal as a prelude to their fusion and partitioning the oronasal chamber.

The transition from vertical to horizontal position is completed within hours. Several mechanisms have been proposed for the rapid elevation of the palatal shelves, including biochemical transformations in the physical consistency of the connective tissue matrix of the shelves; variations in vasculature and blood flow to these structures; a sudden increase in their tissue turgor; rapid differential mitotic growth; an intrinsic shelf force; and muscular movements.

The intrinsic shelf-elevating force is chiefly generated by accumulation and hydration of hyaluronic acid. The alignment of mesenchymal cells within the palatal shelves may serve to direct the elevating forces while palatal mesenchymal cells are themselves contractile. The withdrawal of the embryo's face from the heart prominence by uprighting of the head facilitates jaw opening. Mouth-opening reflexes have been implicated in the withdrawal of the tongue from between the vertical shelves, and pressure differences between the nasal and oral regions due to tongue muscle contraction may account for palatal shelf elevation.

The epithelium overlying the edges of the palatal shelves is especially thickened, and their fusion upon mutual contact is crucial to intact palatal development[55].

Embriological Causes for the Formation of Cleft

According to Ross and Johnson, 1972, most studies on the embryogenesis of the primary palate in man and experimental animals have demostrated that they result from failure of the "epithelial fusion-mesenchymal consolidation" process. They indicate that the cleft may be the result of:

1. Failure of the processes to come in contact
2. Failure of epithelial fusion after contact
3. Failure of mesenchymal consolidation
4. Rupture of the primary palate subsequent to fusion.
5. Reduced facial mesenchyme.
6. Increased facial width.
7. Distortion or malposition of the facial processes.

Chapter-5

ETIOPATHOGENESIS

Anomalies of the face and jaws fall into the sphere of many specialists because they involve different organ systems and functions. To treat these deformities in a rational manner and to gain some understanding of possible methods of prevention, an understanding of the etiology and pathogenesis of malformation is necessary.

Both cleft lip with or without Palate and cleft palate alone are etiologically heterogenous. There is not a single cause or any single etiological model that explains the occurrence of either type of cleft. Single genes, chromosomal disorders or environmental factors may cause clefts.

Genetic Aspect of Etiology:

Early estimates of the genetic contributions to oral facial clefts ranged from about 12% to 20% with the remainder attributed to environmental factors or gene – environmental interactions. Estimates from most recent studies suggest that about 20 to 50% may be more accurate (Murray[103] 1995, and Wyszinski et al[170] 1996).

Less than one fourth of all cases of cleft lip and palate are multiple occurrences in near relatives of a single family (familial cases). The remainders are isolated instances that do not show familial predisposition.

Studies of the cleft lip and palate phenotype in twins indicate that monozygous twins have about 40% concordance, whereas dizygous twins show only a 5% concordance. These two pieces of information give strong evidence for a hereditary basis for the cleft lip and palate trait. It led many researchers to believe that there was a better explanation for clefts that lie in "single mutant gene" model or the 'Major gene' hypothesis

The "Major gene" hypothesis:

For the past three decades, there has been increasing interest in the possibility that many nonsyndromic clefts may actually be caused by a single mutant gene rather than by many unidentified genes acting together.

Some investigators have felt that the patterns of occurrence of cleft lip with or without cleft palate in families' best fit the model of an autosomal recessive gene with reduced penetrance and variable expressivity.

Some current researchers view the multifactorial inheritance model for clefts as something that was useful when geneticists had no other way to predict recurrence of clefts and feel that the need for such a model will gradually diminish as more genes are mapped and identified. However, the multifactorial threshold model is still used in the counseling of the majority of families.

Despite numerous extensive investigations, however, no simple Mendelian pattern of inheritance is readily apparent. This has led to the proposal by different authors of a variety of genetic modes of inheritance including dominance, recessiveness, sex linkage and various modifying conditions such as incomplete penetrance and variable expressivities.

The following statements represent the current thought concerning the hereditary basis for cleft lip and palate:

1)   Cleft lip with or without cleft palate is a different entity from isolated cleft palate.   The latter clefting entity has a different embryologic history and developmental timing, and it appears to be more susceptible to induction by environmental teratogens.
2)   Cleft lip and palate, and cleft palate only can be divided into 3 subgroup.
    a. Syndromes with clefts:

There are cases of children who have clefts plus other major and minor malformations that collectively compose a syndrome. More than 342 syndromes have been found out as having the cleft palate as an intergral feature of the syndrome.
Examples of Syndromes associated with cleft palate:

1. Pierre – Robin syndrome
2. Syndromes associated with the Robin Sequence
    - Stickler syndrome
    - Cerebrocostomandibular syndrome
    - Campomelic syndrome
    - Spondyloepiphyseal dysplasia congenita
    - Persistent left superior vena cava syndrome
    - Myotonic dystrophy
    - Diastrophic dwarfism
    - Donlan syndrome
    - Beckwith–Wiedemann syndrome
    - Radiohumeral synostosis syndrome
    - Partial trisomy 11q. syndrome (and several 'associations')
    - Fetal alcohol syndrome
    - Fetal phenytoin syndrome
    - Fetal trimethadione syndrome
    - Femoral hypoplasia; unusual facies syndrome

3. Treacher collins syndromes
4. Apert syndrome
5. Velocardiofacial syndrome
6. Hemifacial microsomia
7. Mandibulo facial dysostosis
8. Nager syndrome
9. EEC syndrome (Ectodactyly–ectodermal dysplasia–clefting)
10. Frontonasal dysplasia
11. Craniofrontonasal dysplasia
12. Oblique facial clefts
13. Median cleft of the lower lip
14. van der Woude syndrome
15. Cleft palate and ankyloglossia syndrome
16. Down syndrome

So many authors studied some important clefting syndromes elaborately. Rintala et al[123] (1984) and Edwards and Newall (1985) believed that genetically determined disorders in the growth both of the maxila and mandible may result in CP and mircrognathia. Cohen[34] (1982) considered the existence of only a single etiologic or pathogenic agent to be improbable and proposed that the various conditions in which the triad appears, suggested heterogeneity of the etiologic and pathogenic agents. Marques (1998) concluded that heredity could be a factor in the etiopathogenesis of isolated Robin sequence.

Jonathan A. Britto[68] (2002) revealed that the coregulation of molecules of the fibroblast growth factor receptor (FGFR) signaling pathway with transforming growth factor betta3 (TGFbetta3) throughout the stages of human palatal fusion suggests their controlling influence on apoptosis and epithelio mesenchymal transdifferentiation at the Medial Edge Epithelium. Experimental evidence links $FGFG_2$ – Igllla/b loss of function with palatal clefting, and these correlated data suggest a unique pathological mechanism for occurrence of cleft palate in Apert syndrome.

Genetic Aspects of Some Syndromes with Clefting are reviewed in the following table.

Table- 5.1

Syndrome	Gene Map Locus	Comments
van der Woude sysndrome	1q32-q41 17p11.1–p11.2	Autosomal dominant inheritance; gene maps to 1q32 – q41; one large Brazilian family maps to 17p11.1 – p11.2; either the syndrome is genetically heterogenous or the gene at both loci work synergistically, 17p11.1-p11.2 increasing the risk of cleft lip with or without cleft palate.
Treacher Collins syndrome	5q32-q33.1	Treacle gene mutations cause premature termination of the protein

del(22q11.2) syndrome*	22q11.1	Disruption of gene UFD1L alone or in combination with gene CDC45L and / or HIRA has been suggested as the most likely etiology and the role of the dHand-UFD1L pathway have been discussed; however, many patients do not have mutations in these genes. Thus, the genetic etiology is not resolved currently.
X-Linked cleft palate with or without ankyloglossia	(1)Xq21.3-q22 (2)Xq13-q21.31	Genetically heterogenous; (1) is found in German and Icelandic families, (2) is found in British Columbia families.

* Formerly known as Velocardiofacial syndrome, DiGeorge syndrome, or Conotruncal anomalies / Face syndrome.

b. Non-syndromic sporadic cases:

These are isolated occurrences of clefts without other malformations. There is reason to believe that most of these cases are the result of gene environmental interaction and therefore will have little chance to recur in the family.

The first positive association published with oral facial clefts was a population based association between CL / CP and a Tag I restriction site polymorphism in the transforming growth factor alpha (TGFA) locus (Ardinger[6] et al 1989). An association with TGFA has also been reported with CP although most studies of TGFA and CP failed to find an association.

c. Nonsyndromic familial cases:

These familial cases of clefts have a high heritability and although they make up only 10 to 15% of all cleft types, they must be looked for to provide the correct genetic counseling. Inheritance appears to be dominant with incomplete penetrance.

Marazita ML, et al[86] (2002) revealed the Genome scan result for loci involved in cleft lip with or without cleft palate, in Chinese multiplex families. This is the first reported genome-scan study of CL / CP in any Asian population. The following regions had positive multipoint results: chromosomes 1 (90-110 cM), 2 (220-250 cM), 3 (130-150 cM), 4 (140-170 cM), 6 (70-100 cM), 18 (110 cM), and 21 (30-50 cM). The most significant multipoint linkage results were for chromosomes 3q and 4q. Associations with P value of 0 .05 were found for loci on chromosomes 3, 5-7, 9, 11, 12, 16, 20, and 21. The most significant association result (P value of.009) was found with D16S769 (51 cM).

3. The proposed gene for this trait has variable expression, showing itself in one person as a cleft and in another as a soft or hard tissue discrepancy but not a cleft in the clefting area, such discrepancies have been termed "microforms" or incomplete manifestation of gene action.

Examples: Pits of the lip, raphe of lip and bifid uvula. When incomplete manifestations of gene action such as those described are used as evidence for a clefting gene in families, autosomal dominance with decreased penetrance is a reasonable genetic hypothesis for CL with or without CP.

4. Recurrence Risk:

In a recent review of the genetics of cleft lip and cleft palate, Bixler[11] (1981) noted that three subgroups of CL with or without CP and CP only can be recognized. These are designated as (1) syndromic (2) Isolated and (3) familial.

Excluding the small proportion of syndromic cases of clefting, since they have multiple and varied causes, good evidence suggests that the sporadic (single) cases of CL with or without CP and CP only are etiologically different from the familial (multiple) ones.

If the parent is a sporadic case in the family, instead of providing an overall 4% to 5% recurrence risk for that parent's next child, the recurrence risk is about 0.1%. If other family members are also affected this represents a familial case and the recurrence risk is as high as 16%. The following table shows the candidate gene suggested by allelic association and linkage analysis for orofacial clefting.

Table-5.2

Candidate Gene	Gene Map Locus	Name of Gene	Type of Cleft Associated
TGFα	2p13	Transforming growth factor α	CL/CP,CPO
TGFβ	19q13.1-q13.3	Transforming growth factor β	CL/CP
MSX1	4p16.1	Homeobox gene (HOX7)	CL/CP
RARα	17q12	Retinoic acid receptor α	CL/CP
DLX2	2q32	Distal-less homeobox 2	CPO
BCL3	19q13.1	B-cell leukemia / lymphoma 3	CL/CP
	2q32	Unknown gene but different than DLX2; possible candidate genes include FN1, IHH, IGFBP@, and IGFBP5	CPO
	4q25-q31.1	Unknown gene	CL/CP
	6p23	Unknown gene	CL/CP
	17p11.1-p11.2	Unknown gene that may increase cleft palate susceptibility or work synergistically to increase susceptibility in van der Woude syndrome that maps to 1q32-q41	CPO

CL/CP - cleft lip with or without cleft palate, CPO - cleft palate only.

Candidate gene is a gene known to be located in region of interest whose product has biochemical or other properties suggesting that it may prove to be one of the clefting genes sought. Allelic association is joint occurrence of two alleles in a population at a frequency that is greater than expected according to the product of their independent frequencies; the goal is to compare risk factors between a cleft papulation and a defined control group. Linkage analysis is a method to identify whether or not alleles from two loci segregate together in a family.

The Gene-Environment interaction

The gene-environment interaction can be effectively describer by the multifactorial threshould model. Falconer and Carter developed this concept and it has been the most accepted theory for the past several decades.

The "Multifactorial threshold" Model

Most human traits are multifactorial in origin – height, weight, hair colour, eye colour and so on. This means that there are probably several genes, possibly combined with environmental factors that determine the expression of the trait.

The frequency with which the trait is found in the family, and the extent to which it is expressed will depend on sex, degree of relationship, and possibly environmental factors. When a birth defect such as CL with or without CP follows a multifactorial pattern of inheritance,

(1) The affected relatives, if there are any at all, will more likely be first–degree rather than second–degree relatives,
(2) The more severe the defect in the proband, the more likely there will be affected relatives,
(3) The affected relatives will more likely be of the same sex as the proband, and
(4) The more affected relatives there are in the family history, the higher the likelihood of recurrence in future babies.

Schematic portrayal of the multifactorial model:

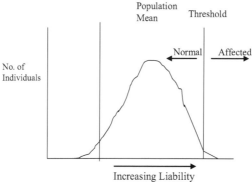

Increasing Liability
No.of genetic and environmental factors

Fig-5.1: It illustrates a population of individuals following the normal population curve with liability for a particular disease, such as cleft lip, increasing to the right.

The multifactorial threshold model depicted in Figure (1) is useful. It shows a theoretical distribution of the genetic and environmental factors for a particular abnormality [e.g., CL/CP] in the general population. The sum of these factors

18

determines the liability of each individual for the abnormalities in that population. If the liability for that individual crosses a threshold (failure of the prominences to contact), the abnormality [CL/CP] would be expressed.

For "rare" abnormalities, the area under the curve (which indicates the number of individuals) beyond the threshold is small. It is virtually impossible to be far beyond (to the right of) the threshold. Thus, the facial prominences of individuals with CL/CP would have barely missed making contact, and slight improvements in the conditions affecting the pregnancy (e.g., elimination of cigarette smoking or the use of vitamin supplements) could substantially improve the chances of contact and prevent an appreciable number of clefts from occurring. The fact that so many clefts are incomplete (when contact is insufficient for complete fusion) indicates that a large number of embryos are sitting squarely on the threshold.

Andrew C. Lindral et al,[5] (1996) carried out studies on the candidate genes $TGFB_2$, MSX_1, TGFA, and $TGFB_3$, in the Etiology of CL /C P in the Philippines. He mentioned that previous association studies using Caucasian populations of nonsyndromic CL/CP and CP only had strongly suggested a role for TGFA in the susceptibility of clefting in humans. Exclusions of significant association in a non-Caucasian population for TGFA suggest that TGFA plays less of a role than it does in Caucasians. This may be due to multiple or different genetic or environmental factors contributing to the etiology of this most common craniofacial anomaly in the Philippine population.

Gary M. Shaw[54] (1997) suggested that infants who have an A_2 TGFA genotype and whose mothers do not use multivitamin containing folic acid periconceptionally are at elevated risk of being born with CL/CP or CP anomalies. This study is among the first to explore the influence of gene-nutrient interactions and its role in formation of orofacial clefts.

Natalie J.Prescott et al.,[104] (2002) evaluated the evidence for the influence of folate genes on craniofacial development. If the FA level in the blood is decreased, there is elevation of plasma homocysteine (a product of folate mebtabolism). Mildy elevated homocysteine has been detected in the blood of mothers with NTD (Neural Tube Defects) pregnancies.

It has been suggested that maternal FA deficiency may, in part be explained by a variant of the 5, 10 methylene tetra hydrofolate reductase enzyme that has a thermolabile variant because of a C to T substitution at position 677, resulting in decreased activity of the enzyme (Kang et al[72] 1991). Homozygosity for this polymorphism has been shown to result in a 7.2 fold increased risk for NTDs and may partially explain why FA prevents this defect in those at increased risk.

One of the most useful metabolic markers for folate deficiency is hyperhomocystinemia and some evidence suggests that this may be a risk factor for oral clefting (Wong et al[166] 1999). Because of the known advantages of folate theraphy during pregnancy and the developmental problems that may occur when diets are folate deficient, recent research has looked toward a possible genetic explanation for susceptibility to low folate states.

Several gene variants have been identified which, when combined with an inadequate diet, may impede human development, but it still remains to be seen whether these are a major contributor to CL / CP.

Environmental Factors:

The environmental factors considered below are selected primarily because there is some evidence of their relevance to CL / CP in humans. Although animal experiments have revealed the contribution of factors and mechanism, how they alter the normal development of lips and palate, none of the factors have been proved to be a sole agent causing this anomaly in human beings.

Most of these factors are yet to be studied in detail, regarding their mechanism of action. Animal experiments showed that these factors contribute in the development of cleft, but they couldn't reveal the exact mechanism of action of each factors in causing cleft lip and palate.

Bronsky et al[23] (1985) revealed the mechanism of action of some environmental factors that inhibit the ETC and effects of hypoxia on facial prominence development in CL/Fr mice. Experimental results from studies on animals showed that environmental factors inhibiting the electron transport chain (ETC)-(Fig.2) were potent inducers of CL / CP in mammals and comparable clefts in chick embryo.

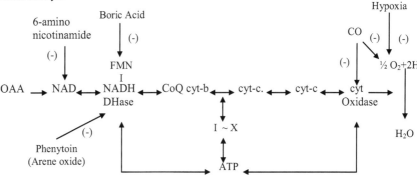

Fig-5.2: Teratogens that block ATP production by interference with electron transport. Elctrons mostly enter the chain via the NAD^+ – NADH dehydrogenase enzyme complex, and as they travel down the chain to progressively lower energy states, ATP is generated. Oxygen is the final acceptor of the electrons.

Disease of mother:

1. Nausea and vomiting in pregnancy.
2. Menstrual disturbances.
3. Viral infections like rubella, measles and cytomegalo virus. Viral infection affecting the mother in the first trimester has more possibility of developing cleft lip and palate in the child.
4. Emotional stress.
5. Hyperthermia during pregnancy: eg. Heat sources like fever etc.
6. Toxemia – Exposure to agricultural and industrial chemicals (Pesticides).
   - Hyper vitaminosis A.
7. Maternal Smoking:

The administration of corbon monoxide (CO) at roughly the same level as that in cigarette smoking (180 ppm) to pregnant A/J mice doubles the incidence of CL/CP (Bailey and Johnston,[8] 1988). Maternal respiratory hypoxia (10 percent O_2 Vs roughly 22 percent in air) dramatically increases the incidence of CL (P) in both CL/Fr mice (Millicovsky and Johnston,[99] 1981; Bronsky, Johnston and sulike, 1986) and A/J mice (Bailey and Johnston, 1988).

Carbon monoxide (CO) blocks electron transport (Fig-5.2) by inhibiting cytochrome oxidase, and also decreases the oxygen supply to tissues by preventing the binding of oxygen to hemoglobin and the release of oxygen from oxyhemoglobin. Hypoxia blocks electorn transport (Fig-5.2) because of the decreased amount of oxygen available to act as the final electron acceptor in this chain of reactions.

The most vulnerable aspect of craniofacial development related to hypoxia appears to be the morphogenetic movement. The principal movements affected are the curling forwards of the lateral portion of the olfactory placode, the bringing together of the median nasal prominences (MNP) in the midline (apparently mediated primarily by forebrain invagination), and the lateral flexure of the distal portion of the MNP. A large amount of cell death is associated with the inhibition of lateral olfactory placodal morphogenesis owing to apparent uncoupling of the terminal web contraction. Edema and minor hemorrhage may also play a role (Grabowski,[57] 1970); however, the authors were unable to find much supporting evidence.

Karin Kallen et al,[76] (1997) revealed the connection between maternal smoking and orofacial clefts. Infants with oral clefts were selected among 1,002,742 infants born between 1983 and 1992 with known smoking exposure in early pregnancy. A statistically significant association with maternal smoking was found.

Diego F. Wyszynski et al[41], (1997) explored the US birth certificates data to estimate the risk of maternal cigarette smoking for oral clefting. This study suggests that smoking during pregnancy is only a minor risk factor for oral clefting in the offspring. He conducted a meta-analysis to estimate the association between maternal cigarette smoking and the risk of having a child with nonsyndromic oral clefts. These

21

analyses suggest a small but statistically significant association between maternal cigarette smoking during the first trimester of gestation and increased risk of having a child with CL and CP.

8.   Alcoholism:

As a positive correlation between smoking and drinking may exist, alcohol could be a confounder of particular interest.

Alcoholism and pregnancy is associated with a pattern of abnormalities in the offspring known as fetal alcohol syndrome (FAS). Clarren and Smith[29] (1978) found that CL/CP occasionally occurred with FAS. More recently Werler et al[162] (1991) estimated the odds ratio for five or more drinks daily among cases of CL and CP to 3.0.

9. Malabsorption Syndromes and Poor Nutrition:

It leads to deficiency of- Vitamin B_1, B_2, B_6, Folic acid, and Vitamin C.

Vitamin B_1
Thiamine was investigated, since a series of authors attributed it with a crucial role in preventing cleft lip, alveolus and palate.

Volker[161] (1996) concluded that, it is of utmost importance that the timing of treatment and dosage of Vitamin B_1 should be taken into consideration not only in animal experiments but also when applying results to humans.

Vitamin B_6
Several clinical studies have shown that Vitamin B_6 therapy can prevent several craniofacial malformations (Conway[35], 1958, Peer et al[109], 1958, 1964).

Catharina Jacobsson et al[25], (1997) studied the effect of Vitamin B_6 on Beta-Aminoproprinonitrile – induced palatal cleft formation in the rat. Apart from clinical studies there are several animal studies showing the preventive effect on craniofacial malformations by Vitamin B_6 (Peer et al 1958, Miller[98], 1972, Dostal and Schubert[42] 1990).

Folic Acid:
Tyan[157], (1982) reported that the frequency of CL with or without CP among Japanese and other Asians born in California and New York was significantly lower than the frequency in the same groups born in Japan and Hawaii; these authors postulated that the effect could be due to better diet. In the early 1980s Tolarova[151] (1982) found evidence that the occurrence of CL with or without CP, as well as other neural tube defects, might be reduced by maternal intake of folic acid. The investigation of folic acid as a factor for reducing occurrence of clefts continues

(Tolarova[150], 1987) and remains one of the few "Proactive" areas of research for helping to eliminate birth defects.

Volker Bienengraber et al[161], (1997) explored the possibility of preventing formation of cleft palate by prenatal administration of folic acid. He described that tetrahydrofolic acid an important coenzyme is formed from folic acid by means of reduction. It is necessary for the biochemical transfer of C_1 – fragments e.g., in amino acid metabolism in general and in DNA synthesis in particular and thus critical for cell proliferation. The folate requirement increases during growth and development of the organs. Hence deficiency of folic acid may result in NTD and oral clefts.

Vitamin C:
Vitamin C is the important factor in the synthesis of collagen fibers in the connective tissues. An interesting observation was provided by the experiments of Landamer and sopher (1970) in which they bypassed the 6-Aminonicotinamide induced block (Fig.2) at the NADH dehydrogenase complex through the use of a high energy intermediate such as ascorbate that donates the electron further down the chain beyond the block. The incidence of 6-AN induced cleft was dramatically decreased. There is some evidence that phenytoin, a potent induces of CL/CP may exert some of its teratogenic activity at the NADH dehydrogenase level.

10. Maternal Metabolic Disease

The role of maternal metabolic disease in the etiology of congenital defects of the head and face is still unclear. Diabetes mellitus has been shown to increase the likelihood of fetal mortality and also to increase the incidence of malformation in the offspring to about three times that found in offspring of non-diabetic mothers. The incidence of facial clefts is much higher in children of mothers with a family predisposition to diabetes.

Drugs
1. Cancer chemotherapeutic agents like Aminopterin, Methotrexate, Cyclophospamide, Procarbazine and Hydroxamic acid derivatives. These drugs interfere with DNA synthesis lead to gross malformation if the fetus survives the abortifacient activity of the drugs.

2. Anticonvulsant drugs such as Phenytoin, Trimethadione, and Paramethadione.These drugs are suspected of causing cleft palate in the offspring of epileptic mothers. The most common drug among the CL / CP inducing environmental factor in which the pathogenesis has been studied is Phenytoin. The incidence of CL / CP in the children of epileptic mothers receiving Phenytoin appears to be approximately ten times that in controls. After treatment of pregnant A/J mice with Phenytoin, the overall growth of the embryo, including the facial prominences, is reduced (Sulik and associates[145], 1979), as reflected by a reduction in the rate of

23

mesenchymal cell proliferation in facial prominences to approximately 50 percent that of controls.

The tissue culture studies of facial prominences revealed that a covering epithelium is necessary for the maintenance of the underlying mesenchyme. It was also noted that growth of the mesenchyme might normally be regulated by epithelial serotonin via the mesenchymal cell process meshwork, which presumably contains the serotonin binding protein found in that area. (Lauder, Tannir and sadler[79], 1988). The anticonvulsant drugs are thought to function therapeutically through interference with neurotransmitters (Serotonin), and it is possible that at least part of their teratogenic activity may result from interference with neurotransmitter regulation of development.

3.   Folic Acid antagonist eg: Mythyl triazene

Frank et al[50] (1989) described the effects of 30 mg/kg of 3.3 dimethyl −1-phenyl triazene administered on day 12 of gestation in the rat.   At external examination, they found 82% of cases with micrognathia and 100% of embryos with CP.

4.   Radiation

Ionising radiation have induced microcephaly and cleft palate in live born offspring whose mothers had been exposed to therapeutic or accidental pelvic radiation during the first ten weeks of pregnancy.

5.   Retinoids

This drug is most commonly used for treatment of cystic acne. It has the teratogenic effect such as abortion, Hydrocephalus and retardation of cell growth.

6.   Other drugs inducing clefts of the palate are,
        Antiemetics, Hydrocortisone analogues, Opioid Drugs,
        Salicylates (Asprin), Diazepam, Boric Acid

7.   6 – Amino Nicotinamide (Nicotinic acid analogue)

Of the environmental factors affecting the NADH dyhydrogenase complex, 6-amino nicotinamide has been the most extensively studied. Where studied, the effects on development appear to be consistent with those resulting from hypoxia.

Social Class

1.   Lower socio economic level   -   Increased incidence of CL/CP
2.   Inadequate prenatal care   -   Maternal health and nutrition

Lower socio economic status is the main causative factor for the occurrence of cleft lip and palate in developing countries like India.

Chapter-6

CLASSIFICATION

Clefts of lip, lip and palate and of palate are classified into three groups. Various classification systems have been proposed, but only a few have found wide clinical acceptance. One of the simplest classifications is the International Classification proposed in 1987, which is ideal for descriptive purposes. Another classification proposed by Kernahan, the 'stippled Y' is more useful for charting clefts in medical records and describing surgery. Incorporating Elsahy's 'peaks' to describe nasal floor involvement in partial clefts has recently extended the simple 'Y'.

1.THE DAVIS AND RITCHE[118] (1922)

Cleft lip and palate cases are divided into three groups (fig. 6.1).
Group I   -   Cleft lip
GroupII   -   Cleft palate
GroupIII   -   Cleft lip and palate
Group I was further subdivided into 1, 2, & 3,

Group I, 1   -   Unilateral cleft lip
Group I, 2   -   Median cleft lip
Group I, 3   -   Bilateral cleft lip

Group II was further divided into 1 and 2

Group II, 1   -   Cleft of uvula and soft palate
Group II, 2   -   Cleft of hard palate

Each of these two subgroups was further divided into 1/3, 2/3, 3/3 cleft depend upon the extend.

Group III was further subdivided into 1, 2, & 3,

Group III, 1   -   Unilateral CL / CP
Group III, 2   -   Median CL / CP
Group III, 3   -   BilateralCL / CP

2. VEAU (1931)

Cleft lip and palate cases are divided into four groups (fig. 6.2).

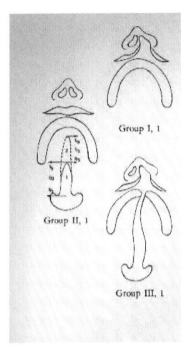

Figure 6.1
The Davis and Ritche Classification

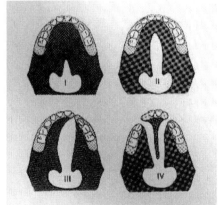

Figure 6.2
The Veau Classification

Group I	-	Clefts of the soft palate
Group II	-	Clefts of the soft and hard palate
Group III	-	Unilateral complete clefts of the alveolus, hard and soft palate
Group IV	-	Bilateral complete clefts of the alveolus, hard and soft Palate

3. FOGH – ANDERSEN (1942)

   1. Harelip (Single or double)

It includes all degrees from a small in the prolabium to a complete cleft of the lip. When thecleft was bilateral through lip and alveolus, he noted, "there is prominence of the premaxilla".

   2. Harelip and cleft palate (Single and double)

He noted complete clefts from nostril to uvula and others broken by osseous and skin bridges.

   3. Cleft Palate

It inlcudes isolated cleft palate and submucous cleft palate.

   4. A group of rare atypical clefts

4. KERNAHAN AND STARK (1958)

   This classification emphasized the embryological basis of the incisive foramen's being set as the boundary marker (fig. 6.3).

1. Clefts of the primary palate
   Cleft lip and pre-maxilla occuring at four to seven weeks of embryonic life

2. Clefts of the secondary palate
   Cefts of the hard and soft palate posterior to the incisive foramen, occuring at 7 to 12 weeks.
   Further descriptions such as left and right, complete and incomplete were added.

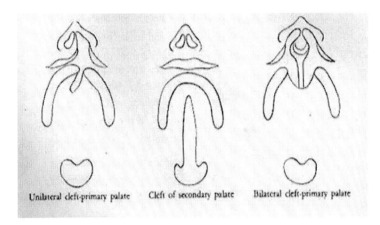

Unilateral cleft-primary palate   Cleft of secondary palate   Bilateral cleft-primary palate

Figure 6.3
The Kernahan and Stark classification

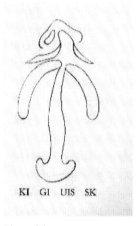

KI GI UIS SK

Figure 6.4
The Vilar-Sancho classification

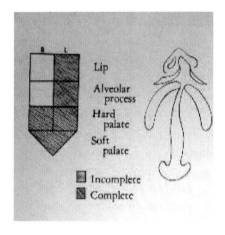

Figure6.5
The Schuchardt classification

28

5. HARKINS (1962)

1.   Cleft of Primary palate
    A)   Cleft lip

      1.   Unilateral: Right, Left
           a) Exten: One third, Two Thirds, complete (1/3, 2/3, 3/3)
      2.   Bilateral: Right and Left
           a) Extent: One third, two thirds, complete (1/3, 2/3, 3/3)
      3.   Median
           a) Extent: One third, two thirds, complete (1/3, 2/3, 3/3)
      4.   Prolabium: Small, Medium, Large
      5.   Congenital scar: Right, Left, Median
           a) Extent: One third, Two thirds, complete (1/3, 2/3, 3/3)

    B)   Cleft of aveolar process
      1.   Unilateral: Right, Left
           a) Extent: 1/3, 2/3, 3/3
      2.   Bilateral: Right, Left
           a) Extent: 1/3, 2/3,3/3
      3.   Median
           a) Extent: 1/3, 2/3,3/3
      4.   Submucous: Riht, Left
      5.   Absent incisor tooth

2.   Cleft of palate
    A. Soft Palate
    1. Posterior: 1/3, 2/3, 3/3
    2. Width: Maximum (mm)
    3. Platal shortness: No, slight, moderate and marked
    4. Smucous cleft
       a) Extent: 1/3, 2/3, 3/3

    B. Hard Palate
    1. Posteroanterior: 1/3, 2/3, 3/3
    2. Width: Maximum (mm)
    3. Vomer attachment: Right, left, absent
    4. Submucous cleft: 1/3, 2/3, 3/ 3

3.   Mandibular Process Clefts
    A. Lip   -   1/3, 2/3, 3/3
    B. Mandible -   1/3, 2/3, 3/3
    C. Lip pits   -   Congenital lip sinuses

4.   Naso-ocular :   Extending from nasial region toward the
                           medial canthal region

5.	Oro-ocular	:	Extending from the angle of the mouth toward the palpebral fissure
6.	Oro-aural	:	Extending from the angle of the mouth.

6. VILAR – SANCHO (1962)

He classified all clefts as incomplete (small letter) or complete (capital) using the appropriate letter of the Greek word (fig.6.4) for the area involved:

K   For kilos   - means lip ⎫
G   For gnato   -   means maxilla ⎪
U   For urano   -   means hard palate ⎬   Location and
S   For Stailos -   means velum ⎪   Extension
⎭

d   for right ⎫
l   for left ⎬   Side
s   for bilateral ⎭

7. SCHUCHARDT (1964)

Visual symbol is used to facilitate indexing cleft lip and palate cases (fig. 6.5).

8. INTERNATIONAL CLASSIFICATION OF CLEFTS OF LIP, ALVEOLUS AND PALATE
(Based on classification suggested at the International Confederation of Plastic Surgeons (1967), modified by the Roger K. Hall[125] (1987) for Group 1 clefts)

Group 1: Clefts of anterior (primary) palate

a. Lip cleft complete
    (a) Lip cleft partial
b. Alveolar cleft including dental lamina
    (b) No alveolar bony cleft but dental lamina involvement, in lateral incisor region beneath lip cleft, as evidenced by the presence of; conical tooth absence of lateral incisor, tooth fusion / germination, enamel hypoplasia of tooth crown and other change in tooth morphology.

Group 2: Clefts of anterior (primary) and posterior (secondary) palate
a. Lip
b. Alveolus
c. Hard palate
d. Soft palate, usually total cleft (if not see below for group 3)

Group 3:   Cleft of posterior (secondary) palate

a. Hard palate
b. Soft palate, degree of partial involvement designated by one-third, two– thirds or submucous.

For all clefts, classification is followed by R (Right), L (Left) or R and L (bilateral). Note : different degrees of clefting may be present on R and L sides.

9. THE 'Y'

Desmound kernahan (1971) found out this classification. As he explained, the bilateral total cleft of the primary and secondary palates can be represented as a Y. The dividing point between the primary and secondary palates – namely, the incisive foramen can be represented symbolically at the junctions of the limbs of the Y by a small circle (fig. 6.6).The right and left limbs of the 'Y' are divided into three sections:

Anterior portion	-	lip (1 and 4)
Middle portion	-	alveolus (2 and 5)
Posterior portion	-	area of hard palate from the alveolus back to incisive foramen (3 and 6)

Posterior to the incisive foramen, the hard (7and 8) and soft (9) palate are also divided into three segments. Rubber stamp can reproduce this segmented Y.
Method:
i)   Stippling the respective segments indicates cleft areas.
ii)   Submucous clefts of the palate are indicated by horizontal lines where a true cleft is not present
iii)   Horizontal lines indicate a simonart's band at the threshold of the nostril across the most anterior portion of the respective limb of the 'Y'.

10.   STRETCHING THE "Y"

Nabil Elsahy (1972) who added triangular peaks (1 and 5) to the ends of the prongs to represent the nasal floor in case of incomplete cleft of the lip (fig. 6.7A&B).

For lip	- 2 and 6
For alveolus	- 3 and 7
For palate anterior to the incisive foramen	- 4 and 8
For hard palate	- 9 and 10
For soft palate	- 11

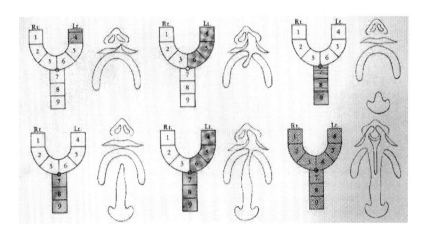

Figure 6.6
The Desmond Kernahan – the 'Y'

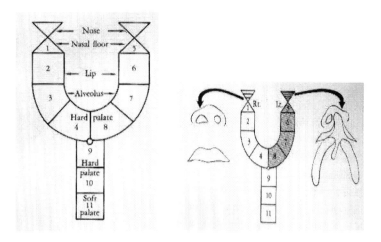

Figure 6.7(A)   Figure.6.7 (B)
The Nabil Elsahy- Stretching the 'Y'   Unilateral Cleft Lip and Palate

32

Vermilion notch	- Stippling in the lower portion of 6th square
Alveolar notch	- Stippling in the upper portion of 7th square
Collapse of maxillary segments	- Stippling or filling in 3 and 4 or 7 and 8
Direction of deflection in complete clefts	- Side of arrow placed lateral to squares 9 and 10
Pharynx	- 12 circle
Velopharyngeal competence	- Dotted line from the Y to12
Premaxilla	- 13 circle
Nasal floor	- 1 and 5
Nose	- Inverted triangle over 1 and 5

11. SPINA (1974)

Group I :   Pre-incisive foramen clefts

    Clefts of the lip with or without alveolar clefts

      a) Unilateral

          i)   right - total when they reach the alveolar arcade or partial

      b) Bilateral

          i)   total

          ii)   Partial   on one or both sides

      c) Median

          i)   total

          ii)   partial

Group II :   Transincisive foramen clefts (Clefts of the lip, alveolus and palate)

      a)   Unilateral   -   right / left

      b)   Bilateral

Group III :   Postincisive foramen clefts

      a)   total

      b)   Partial

Group IV :   Rare facial clefts

12. ORTIZ – POSADAS CLASSIFICATION[107] (2000)

Table – 6.1: Score assigned to the clefts in primary palate

Primary palate	Score
Normal	0
Microform	1
Incomplete 1/3	3
Incomplete 2/3	6
Complete with contact of segments	12

Table –6.2: Factor corresponding to the millimeters of separation of the segments.

Separation (mm)	1	5	10	15	20
Factor	1.1	1.5	2.0	2.5	3.0

Table –6.3: Score assigned to secondary palate clefts

Secondary Palate	Score
Normal	0
Submucous without bifid uvula (soft palate)	1
Submucous with bifid uvula (soft palate)	4
Incomplete 1/3 central (soft palate only)	8
Incomplete 2/3 unilateral (soft palate + one palatal shelf)	13
Incomplete 2/3 bilateral (soft palate + both platal shelves)	14
Complete grade 1* unilateral	25
Incomplete 2/3 + complete grade IIØ	27
Complete grade I bilateral	28
Complete grade II unilateral	34
Incomplete 2/3 + complete grade II	36
Complete grade II bilateral	37
Complete grade III ⊕Unilateral	50
Incomplete 2/3 + complete grade III	53
Complete grade III bilateral	55

* Grade I = Width of palatal shelf greater than width of cleft
ØGrade II = Width of palatal shelf equal to width of cleft
⊕Grade III = Width of palatal shelf less than width of cleft.

METHODS:

Primary Palate:

In order to evaluate their complexity, it was necessary to assign a value to each one of the clefts that may be present. In the care of primary cleft palate, Ortiz-Posadas et al determined together with surgeon that the necessary elements to be considered are:

1. The complexity of unilateral complete clefts without contact between the primary palate segments (cbs).

2. The separation, in millimeters, in the case of unilateral complete clefts without contact between the primary palate segments (wcbs).

3. The additional complexity associated with bilateral clefts.

Scores associated with complexity of unilateral complete clefts with cbs are shown in table –6.1. Scores range from 0 to 12.The degree of seperation between the segments in unilateral complete clefts with no cbs was used to establish level of complexity. The relationship between the magnitude of segment separation and complexity was considered to be directly proportional: the greater the separation, the greater the surgical complexity. As such, a separation factor was assigned to each millimeter of separation (Table–6.2).

Secondary Palate:
In the case of a secondary palate possible clefts and their assigned complexity scores are shown in Table –6.3. The process of assigning these scores was also accomplished jointly with surgeons.

Table –6.4: Features of the lip

Symmetry of lip height	1
Normal lip height	2
Muscular integrity	3
Skin integrity	4
Mucous membrane integrity	5
Symmetry of lip thickness	6
Symmetry of philtral ridges	7
Normal sulcus depth	8
Presence of cupid arch	9

Table –6.5: Features of the Nose

Symmetry of nasal floor	1
Symmetry of nostril arches	2
Symmetry of nostrils (vertical plane)	3
Symmetry of nostrils (antero posterior plane)	4
Nasal septum deviation	5
Length of columella	6
Width of nasal base	7

Lip and Nose:

Various aesthetic features of the lip and nose are incorporated (Table 6.4 and 6.5) into the assessment paradigm. All of the listed features are rated as 'yes'; 'almost' (less than optimal); 'barely' (more deficient); or 'no', with the exception of the length of the columella, which is rated as 'normal'; 'almost' (less than optimal), 'barely', (more deficient); or 'absent' and the width of the nasal base, which is rated as 'greater', 'normal', or 'smaller'.

A mathematical expression was developed to characterize clefts of the primary palate, including the magnitude of palatal segment separation and the added complexity of bilateral clefts, yielding a numerical score that reflects overall complexity of the cleft. Clefts of the secondary palate are also considered in a separate score. Using this method, it is possible to incorporate elements that are not considered in other approaches and to describe all possible clefts that may exist.

Chapter-7

CLINICAL FEATURES

CLEFT LIP

Clinically clefts of the lip vary from a small defect to a complete cleft extending upto and through the floor of the nostril (fig.7.1).

i)   "Microforms" of cleft lip may include a minimal notch in the vermilion, a minor defect where the mucosa of the lip meets the cutaneous portion, a fibrous band or depressed groove running upto the nostril and minor deformity of the nose on the same side.

ii) Microforms of cleft lip have no clinical significance of the speech problems.

iii) A cleft of the lip, even if incomplete, is typically associated with deformity of the nose, causing collapse or flattening on the affected side and a flaring of the alar base.

iv) Cleft lip, defects are often associated with a minor alveolar deformity. A minimal defect of the lip with or without minimal defect of alveolus may also be called as "forme fruste".

v)   There may be a partial bridge of soft tissue across a cleft of the lip and alveolus. It is very thin bridge of soft tissue and is termed as "simonart's band".

vi) Cleft lip is usually, but not always, accompanied by a cleft of the alveolus or dental arch. A complete cleft through the alveolus can extend as far posteriorly as the region of the incisive foramen. The cleft in the alveolus may be minimal or it may extend completely through the arch.

vii) If there is bilateral complete cleft of the lip and alveolus, the central portions of the upper lip and alveolus are attached to the tip of the nose with little or no columella, the strip of tissue between the base and tip of the nose.

viii) Unilateral or bilateral clefts of the lip and alveolus are more often than not associated with clefts of the secondary palate, although there are cases of clefts of the lip and alveolus with no involvement of the secondary palate.

ix) In the unilateral cleft lip, there is a shortening of the lip at the cleft. The vermilion border continues up the cleft margin almost to the nasal floor. The usual orbicularis oris sphincter is broken and it therefore passes upward to become abnormally inserted, mostly into the maxillae around the pyriform aperture either at the alar base or to the anterior nasal spine.

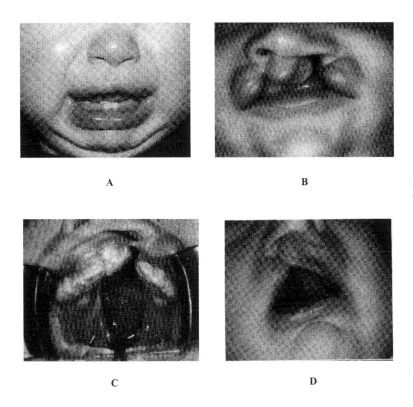

A   B

C   D

Figure. 7.1 Various types of cleft lip   (A) Microform,   (B) Bilateral cleft lip,
                                          (C) Simonart's Band   (D) Unilateral cleft lip

The normal philtrum of the upper lip consists of two parallel vertical ridges largely formed from the depressor septi muscles, these being usually partially present in the unilateral cleft, but missing in the bilateral cleft. The lip on the non-cleft side protrudes further than the lip on the cleft side.

x)   In bilateral cleft lip cases, the defects of both the sides may be symmetrical or asymmetrical (eg. Complete on one side and incomplete on the other side).

xi)   In the bilateral cleft, the orbicularis oris muscle fibres are similarly inserted into the alar base area, but the prolabium, being isolated from the lip musculature, contains few if any muscle fibres. The probabium, which is short and protruded, contains a portion of alveolus and appears to arise from just below the nasal tip – the columella being very short. If there is soft tissue bridging in the submucous type incomplete bilateral cleft, the muscle fibres will tend to fan out through the bridges, but function is grossly impaired.

UNILATERAL CLEFT LIP AND PALATE

Unilateral cleft lip and palate consistently shows an associated skeletal deformity, of which the prominent features are lateral displacement of the noncleft maxillopremaxillary part of the upper jaw, malformation of the nose, and lateral distortion of the nasal septum (fig. 7.2).

1) Premaxillary Segment and Nasal Septum:

The premaxillary segment, in frontal view, tilts upward into the cleft. The interpremaxillary suture is also rotated markedly, as seen in coronal sections, a finding that indicates that the upturning of the premaxillary segment is due to bodily rotation of the entire segment and not solely to a local alveolar deficiency.

The cartilaginous nasal septum is very much bent laterally and upward with the noncleft segment, to which it is attached in the region of the anterior nasal spine. The incisor teeth within the uptilted premaxillary segment later erupt with their crowns tilted and their occlusal plane sloping upward into the cleft. In an older patient, this malocclusion indicates persistence of the original skeletal deformity present at birth.

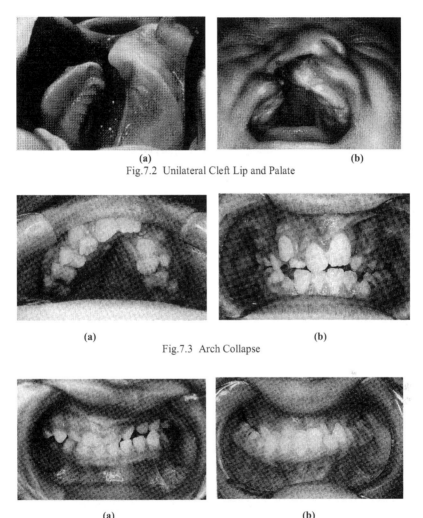

(a)   (b)
Fig.7.2 Unilateral Cleft Lip and Palate

(a)   (b)
Fig.7.3 Arch Collapse

(a)   (b)
Fig.7.4 Dental Maloclusions in Unilateral Cleft Lip and Palate

The deviated nasal septum and displaced premaxillary region have significant implications with regard to the height of the middle third of the face. In cases with unilateral cleft lip and palate, there is often a lateral crossbite on the side of the cleft that is the lateral segment of the maxilla is positioned medialy to its counterpart in the mandible. This is termed "arch collapse" (fig.7.3).

In some children the malrelationship between the maxillary and mandibular teeth may be confined only to the teeth nearest the cleft, not affecting the rest of the dental arch, so that the molar relationship is in fact normal whereas in other children the entire lateral segment is medial to the teeth in the mandible (fig. 7.4).

2) Lip and Columella:

The lip over the premaxillary segment is subjected to a unilateral muscle pull, which tends to retract it from the gingival pad over the incisor tooth of the cleft side, thus contributing to lip distortion. The latter finding can be attributed to the fact that the muscle band of the orbicularis oris inserts at the border of the cleft along the vermilion border, which turns superiorly at the cleft.

A columella may be identified in relation to the noncleft nostril, but on the cleft side, it is merged with the stretched ala nasi. The columellar skin is more developed than in the bilateral cleft condition, but the deviated nasal septum and asymmetric alar cartilages jeopardize the prospects of normal development of a symmetric columella and adequate support for the nose.

Palatal Process and Vomer:

In the secondary palate the cleft may be unilateral or bilateral with respect to the nasal septum. In non-cleft cases; it is symmetrically attached to the inferior border of the septal cartilage, tending to thin laterally in later infancy to develop a sharp inferior edge.

In either case (unilateral or bilateral), since the deformity of the primary palate is similar, the middle third of the nasal septum distends into the nasal cavity corresponding to the side of the cleft lip. In the event of unilateral union between the nasal septum and a secondary palatal process, the nasal floor thus formed is stretched laterally.

The noncleft maxilla is displaced away from the cleft, the cartilaginous septum is distended into the nasal cavity on the cleft side, and the horizontal palatal process is stretched so that the vomer is pulled into the nasal floor.

At birth, both nasal cavities are functionally obstructed -the noncleft side anteiorly at the nostril, and the cleft side posteriorly at the conchal level.

Periodontal problem:

Guntler Schultes et al[59] 1998 studied the comparision of periodontal disease in patients with clefts of palate and patient with unilateral clefts of lip, palate and alveolus.

His study showed the prevalence of poor oral hygiene, calculus deposition, and gingival bleeding problems in unilateral cleft lip and palate and alveolus patients. He concluded that patients with unilateral CL/CP and alveolus showed extensive periodontal lesions in maxillary anterior region in contrast to the patients with cleft palate only and also the general population.

BILATERAL CLEFT LIP AND PALATE

The complete bilateral cleft at birth shows a distinct premaxillary malformation characterized by a protrusion of the entire premaxillary bone with respect to the cartilaginous nasal septum and a protrusion of the tooth-bearing alveolar process. The protrusive premaxillary bone obliterates the columellar area of the nose so that the lip attches directly to the nasal tip.

The total protrusion seen clinically is the summation of three factors: the abnormal forward position of the premaxillary alveolar bone, an abnormally advanced position of the premaxillary basal bone, and possible underdevelopment of the maxillary segments as a whole, including some degree of anteriorly localized hypoplasia at the site of the canine tooth (fig. 7.5).

In bilateral clefts, there is bilateral crossbite, meaning collapse of both arches in the maxilla. It may also occur in unilateral clefts, particularly when there are congenitally missing teeth.

In bilateral cleft palate cases, the premaxilla may vary in size and development and it is seperated from maxilla by the cleft. It may contain the four-insisor teeth often only one or two teeth are present, and occasionally a supernumerary or a normal tooth may be encased in a saclike structure protruding from one side of the premaxilla.

The maxillary process lacking attachment to the premaxilla and not influenced by the growing septal cartilage may appear small and retruded.

If the premaxilla is positioned behind the mandibular teeth there may be a crossbite or class III malocclusion. In some cases the premaxilla may still be positioned anteriorly (in front of the mandibular teeth), with the lateral segment collapsed behind it (fig. 7.6 a).

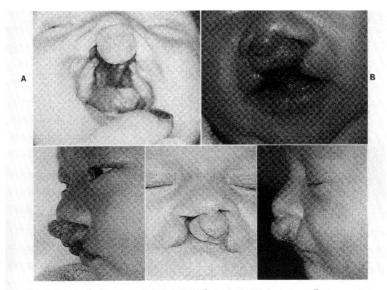

Fig.7.5 A to E, prominent, anteriorly displaced premxilla in infants with complete bilateral cleft lip, with absence of the columella of the nose

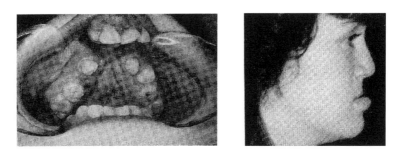

(a) premaxillary protrusion   **(b) Class III Pattern**

Fig.7.6 Bilateral Cleft Lip and Palate

Mandibular prognathism occurs in most cases of cleft lip and palate disorder. But mandibular retrognathism also occurs in some frequency, noted by Bindler and Hopkin (1963). In Pierre Robin syndromic patients, cleft lip and palate is associated with retrognathic mandible, maxillonasal dysplasia and also resultant respiratory problems.

In normal structure the alveolar process is directly inferiror to the basal bone, but in the bilateral cleft condition, the alveolar bone is anterior to the basal bone in horizontal arrangement.

The basal bone and the anterior nasal spine normally lie posterior to the anteroinferior point of the nasal septum, whereas the basal bone of the bilateral cleft premaxillae is anteriorly advanced and adapted around this septal point, and the anterior nasal spine ascends the anterior septal border.

In profile view the primary central incisor teeth lie anterior to the cartilaginous nasal septum. The incisors are not rotated forward and upward, as might be thought, but have a relatively normal vertical orientation. They are supported by a thin protruding alveolar process, which commences at the level of the anterior nasal spine, passes forward over the developing incisor roots, inferior to the medial crura of the alar cartilages, and turns inferiorly for a short distance in relation to the labial surface of the teeth.

1) Lip and Columella:

Labial muscle fibers insert densely, into the skin lateral to the philtrum, which, not receiving such support, presents the median philtral dimple.The medial part of the bilaterally cleft upper lip is conspicuously everted.

The eversion of the lip and to some extent, the hypoplasia of the columellar skin appears to be caused by the premaxillary protrusion. The columella may be clinically absent, but it is not anatomically absent.

2) Nasal Septum, Premaxilla, and Vomer:

In the bilateral cleft condition, the inferior border of the cartilaginous nasal septum is reinforced by bone, which provides a stemlike support for the premaxillary segment. This stem consists mainly of the vomer, its anterior part being formed by the premaxilla.

The premaxillovomeral joint is located at a point approximately one-third of the septal length posterior to the premaxillary alveolar process. The premaxillary segment consists of paired premaxillary bones joined in the midline by the interpremaxillary suture, which represents the anterior third of the normal midpalatal suture.

Posteriorly the premaxillary stem consists of paired processes joined by the suture and termed the infravomerine processes of the premxilla. These overlap the single vomer, whose tapering anterior edge adapts closely to the nasal septum.

The vomer adapts to the inferior border of the cartilaginous nasal septum and articulates posteriorly with the sphenoid bone. In cross section the vomer of prenatal specimens is "U" shaped, but after birth resorption occurs on its lateral surfaces to give a thin "V" shaped cross section with a notable edge inferiorly.

A slight swelling frequently occurs on the inferior border of the septum just posterior to the alveolar process at a position corresponding with the location of the premaxillovomer suture.

CLEFT PALATE

A cleft of the secondary palate involves both the hard palate and the soft palate form the uvular processes posteriorly to the junction with the primary palate anteriorly; the junction corresponds with the position of the incisive foramen on an intact skull. It may range from minimal defects to complete defect extending all the way forward to the region of the incisive foramen (fig. 7.7).

When clefts of the secondary palate, particularly small ones, occur without clefts of the lip and alveolus, they are less likely to be detected in the immediate postnatal period unless the baby is having problems in feeding.

Clefts of the hard palate can be devided into following subtypes;

i)   "Minimal defects"
Here the defect of the palate is as small as a slight scallop or streak in the uvula.

ii)   "Bilateral defects"
Technically, a complete cleft of the secondary palate is termed "bilateral" when both the palatine shelves have not fused with the vomer bone in the superior surface.

iii)   Complete unilateral cleft lip and palate.
This term is given to the cleft extend through the lip, alveolus and anterior section of the hard palate combined with a complete cleft of the secondary palate

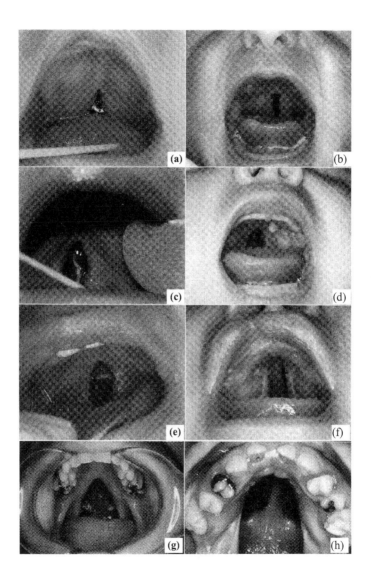

Fig.7.7 Cleft Palate

Submucous clefts of the secondary palate:

There may be significant defects of the hard palate in the absence of an actual opening into the nasal cavity. Classic submucous cleft palate is characterized by a relatively well-defined clinical triad, which results in failure of complete soft palate closure, velopharyngeal insufficiency and hypernasal speech pattern (fig.7.8).

Samuel Stal et al[132] 1998, revealed the clinical feature of classic and occult submucous cleft palate. Although classic submucous cleft palate may be diagnosed based upon a thorough clinical examination and endoscopic examination of superior aspect of the soft palate. Occult submucous cleft palate may display only muscle malposition and hypernasal speech without overt physical findings (fig. 7.9).

This structural abnormality reflects that the musculature of soft palate in particular, the musculus uvulae and levator vali palatini inserts on to the palatine bone rather than forms an adequate muscular sling and palatine aponeurosis. Several types of occult submucous cleft palate have been defined based on anatomic defects noted on surgery.

Features of classic submucous cleft palate:

Triad of overt physical findings
1)   Bifid uvula
2)   Furlow along midline of soft palate
        a. Attenuated midline raphe
        b. Short palate with midline muscle seperation.
3)   Notch in posterior margin of hard palate.

Functional findings in classic SCP:

1)   Hyper nasal speech
2)   Velopharyngeal insufficiency
        a. Aberrant insertion of levator veli palatini upon osseous posterior aspect of palatine shelves.
        b. Failure to form a muscular sling across midline.
        c. Abnormalities in musculature and supporting tissues.

Features of Occult SCP

Muscle malposition in the absence of overt physical findings.
Hypernasal resonance during speech.
Small central gaps in velopharyngeal sphincter during velopharyngeal competency evaluation.

Types of occult SCP
It is classified according to muscle malposition determined at surgery.

Type A

a)   Notched midline posterior palatine shelf
b)   Major portion (75% - 90%) of muscular inserts into posterior palatine shelf.
c)   Some musculature meets at midline
d)   Minimal muscular soft palate sling
e)   Lacks soft palate aponeurosis

Type B

a)   Flat midline posterior palatine shelf.
b)   Moderate position of musculature inserts into posterior palatine shelf.
c)   Moderate muscular soft palate sling.
d)   Lacks soft palate aponeurosis.

Type C

a)   Bifid midline posterior palatine shelf.
b)   Minimal portion of musculature inserts into posterior palatine shelf.
c)   Nearly complete muscular soft palate sling.
d)   Lacks soft palate aponeurosis.

Additional association with SCP and occult SCP

Facial features:

1)   Maxillary hypoplasia (75% dish face)
2)   Lip contour deformity along vermillion border (75% , gull wing)
3)   Oral commisure laxity (25%)
4)   Facial musculature dysfuction (25%)
    a. Horizontal paranasal bulge
    b. Vertical lateral lip bulge
    c. Lack of facial expression
5)   Superior helix with flat arc (10%)
6)   Alveolar arch abnormalities (5%)

Decreased hard palate length
Increased naso pharyngeal depth
Decreased soft palate length.

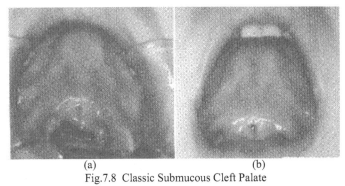

(a)   (b)
Fig.7.8 Classic Submucous Cleft Palate

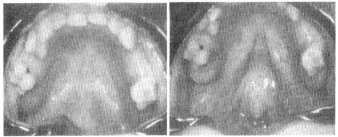

Fig.7.9 Occult Submucous Cleft Palate

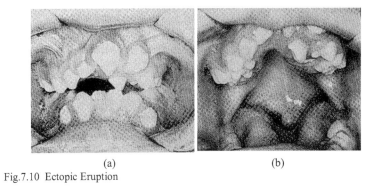

(a)   (b)
Fig.7.10 Ectopic Eruption

COMMON FEATURES

. 1) Facial Appearance

Hopkin (1963) and Bindler (1962), suggested the facial appearance at birth resembled archinencephaly. The absent or rudimentary anterior nasal spine with resulting abnormal nasolabial muscle attachments give rise to the acute nasolabial angle and convex upper lip. This reduced midface prominence gives the appearance typical of the anomaly with a concave profile (fig. 7.6 b).

Hypoplasia of the middle third of the face associated with congenital absence of the anterior nasal spine and Bindler in 1962 and Hopkin in 1963 described depression of the nasal bones with flattened nasal alae.

In the older child with an unrepaired unilateral cleft, there is an increase in facial width probably due to the loss of normal facial muscle action and the action of the tongue and cheek muscles and also palatal shelf growth is distorted by the tongue.

2) Defects of Tooth Formation in Cleft Dentitions

A number of defects of tooth development occur with increased frequency in children with cleft lip and palate. Fifteen different types of abnormality have been listed. The main anomalies in clefts of lip and palate in the Royal Children's Hospital Series were:

- Supernumerary teeth: 41 per cent
- Congenitally missing teeth: 39.4 per cent
- Abnormal crown form or conoid, lateral incisor teeth (other than supernumerary teeth): 4.7 per cent
- Geminated and fused teeth: 1.8 per cent.

Supernumerary Teeth:

In almost all cases, a lateral incisor tooth of normal crown form in the region of the cleft is absent, being replaced by one or more supernumerary teeth (usually conical or conoid). These are frequently erupted at birth as natal teeth high in the cleft labialy in some cleft of lip with no apparent involvement of the alveolus; a geminated, fused or supernumerary tooth is frequently present in the lateral incisor position beneath the cleft lip.

In addition, mainly in cleft lip (but also in clefts of lip and palate), a geminated or conical tooth may be present on the non-cleft side, in the lateral incisor region possibly representing the mildest "forme fruste" of the clefting process in the lip/alveolus region.

Crown Form Abnormalities:

A total of 15 consistently seen abnormalities of dental development have been recorded in patients with clefts. These are:

1. Thick curved maxillary incisors
2. Excess mammelons
3. Exaggerated mammelons
4. Supernumerary teeth
5. Missing teeth
6. Peg-shaped (conoid) incisors
7. T-shaped lateral incisors
8. Malformed mandibular first primary molars
9. Malformed maxillary first primary molars
10. Missing hypocone
11. Reduced hypocone
12. Fused protocone and metacone
13. Malformed mandibular bicuspids
14. Irregular mammelons
15. Labial tubercles
16. Ectopic teeth (fig. 7.10)

The main crown form abnormalities of central incisors and supernumerary teeth adjacent to the cleft and lateral incisors on the non-cleft side have been classified as:

1. T-cingulum teeth
2. Peg-shaped (conical) teeth
3. Thick -curved hypoplastic incisors
4. Marked incisal edge notching of incisors

Developmental Enamel Defects (Hypoplasia and Opacity defects):

These defects of the incisors and/or supernumerary teeth adjacent to the cleft are extremely common in both primary and permanent dentitions (approximately 60 per cent of permanent central incisors were affected in cleft of the lip and palate) such defects arise mainly as a result of the biological clefting process and consequent dental lamina cellular disruption in utero.

Studies on Dental Problems:

1) Alexandra Sarzyla Medeiros et al[1] in 2000, studied the prevalence of intranasal ectopic teeth in children with complete unilateral and bilateral cleft lip and palate. The prevalence of an intranasal tooth for the whole group was 0.48 % and it appeared to be more common in females.

2)   Zhuan Bian et al[172] in 2001, studied the caries experience and oral health behavior in Chinese children with cleft lip and plate. The results of that study show that

   i)   Children with a CL /P have higher levels of dental caries compared to those with a cleft lip alone;

   ii)   The two most important factors for dental caries were:

      a)   whether the child had been bottle – fed and;

      b)   the educational attainment level of the mother.

3.   Jaksi D N et al[66], in 2002 studied the mesiodistal size of deciduous teeth in subjects with unilateral cleft lip and palate. A difference between the genders was found. In the sample of boys the lateral deciduous incisors and the second deciduous molars on the cleft side were smaller than those on the non-cleft side, while in girls the central and lateral deciduous incisors were smaller on the cleft side than on the non-cleft side.

3) Ear Problem:

   i) Hearing loss occurs in 50% of cleft patients this is being caused by functional abnormalities of the pharyngotympanic tubes.

   ii) Accumulation of serous fluid in the middle ear is common. It may result in serous otitis media. It may lead to suppurative otitis media.

   iii) Children afflicted with a cleft of the soft palate are predisposed to middle ear infections. Chronic serous otitis media is common among children with CL and CP and it is associated with hearing loss.

   iv) The type of hearing loss experienced by the patients with CL / CP is conductive, meaning that the neural pathway to the brain remains functioning normally. The defect in these instances is simply that the sound cannot reach the auditory sensory organ as efficiently as it should because of the chronic inflammatory changes in the middle ear. However, if the problem is not corrected, permanent damage to the auditory sensory nerves can also result.

   v) In some associations or syndromes, there is a known risk of sensorineural or mixed hearing loss. Eg. Stickler syndrome and Velocardiofacial syndrome. But most of the syndromes with ear disease show the tendency of resulting in conductive loss. Eg. Robin sequence, mandibulo facial disostosis, Nager syndrome, Apert syndrome, Crouzon syndrome and Pfeiffer syndrome.

vii) Complications of untreated serous otitis media:

Tympanic membrane perforations, cholesteatomia, ossicular chain discontinuity and fixation, mastoiditis, labyrinthitis, and infections of the auditory canal and decreased pneumatization of temporal bone. (Stool and Winn in 1969).

4) Oronasal Fistulae:

Communication between oral and nasal cavities can occur in both cleft lip and palate and cleft palate only cases. Fistulae can occur in the following locations and scenarios:

1. Unoperated, open pathways into the nasal cavity through the labial sulcus and alveolus.
2. Intentionally unrepaired or postsurgical fistulae in the anterior portion of the hard palate primarily in the region of the incisive foramen (left open because the original cleft was so large that the surgeon did not attempt complete closure or fistulae that opened spontaneously after surgery).
3. Fistulae opening spontaneously after surgery at the juncture of the hard and soft palate.
4. Fistulae in the soft palate itself.
In addition any combination of these defects is possible.

Problems associated with oronasal fistulae are:
     i.   Difficulty in feeding
     ii.   Drainage of nasal secretions into the oral cavity
     iii.   Speech problems

The effects on speech will be dependent at least in part on the size of the opening, the location, and the developmental time in the child's acquisition of communication skills in which the fistula is or was present.

5) Feeding Problems:

i. Babies with cleft palate can swallow normally once the material being fed reaches the hypopharynx but have extreme difficulty in producing the necessary negative pressure in their mouth to allow sucking either breast or bottle milk.

ii. When a nipple is placed in the baby's mouth, he or she starts to suck just like any other newborn, because the sucking reflexes and swallowing reflexes are normal. However the musculature is underdeveloped or not properly oriented to allow the sucking to be effective.

SECONDARY DEFORMITIES

Secondary deformities can exist after repair of cleft lip or cleft lip and palate and can affect some or all of the previously cleft regions. There may be lip distortion, nasal deformity, and maxillary hypoplasia; the alveolus may be partly edentulous; and there may be malocclusion, fistula, and palatal dysfunction. The degree of the deformities is usually related to several variables: the severity of the original defect, the method of repair and subsequent healing, the inherent and familial patterns of the patient's craniofacial growth, the effectiveness of orthodontic therapy, and the adequacy of prosthetic rehabilitation.

Lip Deformities:

1. Lip scars - It is unavoidable from any techniques.

2. Long lip - Due to techniques of Le Mesurier (1949),
   Tennison (1952) and Ramdall (1959). It can also occur as a result of the rotation advancement lip repair owing to excessive rotation (millard 1974, Bardach and Salyer, 1987).

3. Short lip (vertical deficiency) – It occurs due to vertical scar contracture.
   (Bardach and salyer 1987)
4. Tight lip (horizontal deficiency) – Due to sacrifice of excessive soft tissues during the primary lip repair.
5. Orbicularis oris abnormalities- Inadequate muscle reconstruction results in a lip that functions improperly in speech, facial expression, whistling and mastication.
6. Lip Landmark abnormalities.
   i) Loss of philtral definition
   ii) Obliteration of the Cupid's bow
   iii) Vermilion deficiency. – Whistle Deformity
   The most common secondary deformity of the vermilion in unilateral cleft lip is deficiency of the Cupid's bow. This may be verticle in orientation with a notching deformity of the vermilion, a mismatch of the vermilion margins, or an attenuated or absent vermilion ridge. It is known as whistle deformity.

7. Deficient buccal sulcus:
   A shallow buccal sulcus is unusual in unilateral cases but commonly occurs in the prolabial area in bilateral clefts.

Nasal Deformities:

1. The tip of the nose is deflected toward the noncleft side.
2. The dome on the cleft side is retrodisplaced.

3. The angle between the medial and lateral crura on the cleft side is excessively obtuse.
4. The alar buckles inward on the cleft side.
5. The alar-facial groove on the cleft side is absent.
6. The alar – facial attachment is at an obtuse angle.
7. There is real or apparent bony deficiency of the maxilla on the cleft side.
8. The circumference of the naris is greater on the cleft side.
9. The naris on the cleft side is retrodisplaced.
10. The columella is shorter in the antero–posterior dimension on the cleft side.
11. The medial crus is displaced on the cleft side.
12. The columella is positioned obliquely, with the dorsal ends slanted toward the non – cleft side.
13. Nasolabial fistula.
14. Absence of the nasal floor.
15. Hypertrophy of the interior turbinate on cleft side.
16. Displacement of the noncleft maxillary segment.
17. Vestibular web – a characteristic linear contracture of the interior nostril from its apex to the piriform aperture along the upper border of the alar cartilage. This is due to anteroposterior shortness of the maxilla.

Not all deformities are present in each patient, nor are they present to the same degree.

Maxillary Deformities:

1. Maxillary retrusion
2. Collapse of maxillary segments

Palatal Deformities:

1. A frequent incidence of oronasal fistula after primary palatal repair.
2. A greater deficiency of bony and soft tissue.
3. A protruded premaxilla from the midline.
4. Persistent mobility of the premaxilla.

Palatal Fistula:
The most common defect in the hard palate after repair is the fistula (Stal and Spina, 1984). It may be located anterior or posterior to the alveolar ridge. Fistulas occur more frequently after palatoplasty for complete clefts of the primary and secondary palates (CL/CP) than after that for isolated secondary palate clefts (CP)

Alveolar Clefts:

A residual alveolar defect associated with an oronasal fistula has many sequelae (Waite and Kesten, 1980).

Most commonly occuring secondary alvelor defects are:
1.   Tooth malposition
2.   Oronasal air escape
3.   Facial asymmetry

SPEECH PROBLEMS:

Alterations in resonance:

1.   Hypernasality
2.   Hyponasality
3.   Mixednasality
4.   Cul-de-sac

Hypernasality:

Hypernasality is a resonance alteration of vowels and vocalic consonants that occurs when the oral and nasal cavities are abnormally coupled. The result is that the sound wave is diverted into the nasal airways. And speech sounds as if it is coming through the nose.

Hyponasality:

Hyponasality refers to a reduction in nasal resonance that is heard when the nasal airway itself is partially blocked or the entrance to the nasal passages is partially occluded, as might occur if a moderately large adenoid pads were present. If the nasal airways were completely occluded, speech would be denasal, meaning that nasal airflow associated with /m/, /n/, and /η/, would be eliminated and the sound wave altered; the nasal consonants would approach but not match /b/, /d/, and /g/.

Mixed nasality:

A number of authors (Mc Williams and Philips, 1990; Peterson-Falzone, 1982) have described resonance characterized by elements of both hyponasality and hypernasality. Hypernasality and hyponasality may co-occur in patients with velophamgeal inadequacy who evidence increased nasal resistance that is not great enough to eliminate nasal resonance entirely but is too great to permit nasal consonants to maintain their integrity. This resonance pattern is more frequently perceived in patients with a pharyngeal flap or prosthetic devices.

Cul – de sac:

Cul–de–sac resonance is a variation of hyponasality. It differs only in the place of obstruction and in the way the speech sounds. A cul-de-sac is defined as a blind pouch or a passage with only one outlet. The speech has a muffled characteristic.

Articulation disorders:

1. Nasal emission.
2. Inaudible nasal emission.
3. Audible nasal emission.

Nasal emission:

Hypernasality and nasal emission are both speech characteristics associated with poor velopharyngeal structure and function. Although hypernasality is a resonance disorder that influences the character of vowels, nasal emission is an articulation disorder that affects high – pressure consonants. Nasal emission of air may be associated with reduced oral air pressure for pressure consonants, and the combination of hypernasality and reduced oral breath pressure may mask place and manner of articulation.

Inaudible nasal emission:

Normally, most speakers produce connected discourse without evidence of nasal air escape. Speakers who do not achieve sufficient velopharyangeal closure for production of the pressure sounds may demonstrate visible nasal escape from one or both nostrils for obstruents.

Audible nasal emission:

Audible nasal emission can be defined as the sound that is heared when air passes through the nasal passages. You can create audible nasal emission by exhaling forcibly through your nose. This rush of air creates a noise that becomes a part of the speech signal generated and influences how it is preceived by listeners. When marked intranasal resistance to airflow is present, the speech sound may be accompanied by extraturbulent noises, which we refer to as nasal turbulence (McWilliams[91], 1982).

Morley[102] (1970) referred to a "nasopharyngeal snort' that results from the passage of air through a sphincter that is closed but not tightly so. Although velopharyngeal closure may be sufficient for impounding intraoral air pressure for obstruents, these consonants may be released nasally rather than orally. This may reflect weak closure of the velopharyngeal port. Morley stated that these snorts often accompany /s/ sounds and other fricatives but can be associated with other sounds as well.

McWilliams and Musgrave (1977) warned that other speech disorders, such as lateralized /s/ associated with dental anomalies, may easily be confused with audible nasal emission and attributed mistakenly to a faulty valve. This occurs because both types of errors are associated with an alteration in the direction of the air stream for speech but for different reasons.

Compensatory articulation patterns:

Atypical patterns of articulation have often been observed in the speech of individuals with cleft palate. Some of these patterns appear to develop in compensation for velopharyngeal inadequacy, whereas others develop in compensation for palatal fistulae or malocclusion.

Glottal stops:

Glottal stops are the most common compensatory articulations produced by individuals with cleft palate (Peterson-Falzone[110], 1989; Trost – Cardamone[153], 1990). These laryngeal productions typically occur as substitutions for oral stop consonants but are also frequently substituted for fricatives and affricates.

Pharyngeal fricatives:

Pharyngeal fricatives are produced as turbulent air passes through a constriction created by the tongue dorsum and posterior pharyngeal wall (Morley[102]. 1970; Trost[156], 1981). These linguopharyngeal productions are typically substituted for oral fricatives and affricates but may also occur as co–articulations (Henningsson and Isberg[62], 1986; Trost 1981). Morley (1970) distinguished between pharyngeal and glottal fricatives. The former involved use of frication between the tongue dorsum and the pharyngeal wall, whereas the latter is "made with increased frication between overtense vocal cords". Pharyngeal fricatives are rare other than in the speech of persons with cleft palate or related conditions.

Laryngeal fricative:

The laryngeal fricative was produced with a constriction formed by the depressed epiglottis and the elevated arytenoid cartilages. Trost – Cardamone (1997) asserted that the laryngeal fricative is probably not a "categorically distinct" compensatory articulation but instead appears to be a variant of the pharyngeal fricative.

Additional compensatory patterns of articulation have been described in recent years, including the pharyngeal stop, Pharyngeal affricate, posterior nasal fricative, velar fricative, palatal fricative, and the middorsum palatal stop. The pharyngeal stop was described as a linguopharyngeal stop substitution for /k/ and /g/. Trost noted that the location of this stop is influenced by the phonetic context in which it occurs. Trost – cardamone[153] (1990) has since described the pharyngeal affricate an articulatory gesture that consists of both a glottal stop and a pharyngeal affricate

Posterior nasal fricative

The posterior nasal fricative is produced as the velum approximates the posterior phyaryngeal wall but leaves an incompletely closed velopharyngeal port. According to Trost[156] (1981) the posterior nasal fricative is distinctive because of audible frication. It is typically substituted for /s/, /z/, /ʃ/, /3/ and may as a co-articulation with fricatives, affricates, or stop consonants. Posterior nasal fricatives are frequently the predominant misarticulation observed in patients with phoneme-specific nasal emission and have also been observed in patients after pharyngeal flap surgery.

Middorsum palatal stop

The third type of articulation described by Trost (1981) was a middorsum palatal stop. The place of articulation for this stop production is similar in vocal tract location to that used for /j/. When used, it occurs as a substitution for /t/, /d/, /k/, or /g/.

Velar Fricative

The velar fricative has been described as a compensatory gesture produced when air flows through a constriction created between the tounge dorsum and velum. It can be thought of as a /k/ produced as a fricative. It typically occurs as a substitution for oral fricatives or velar stops (Bzoch, 1956; Lynch, Fox, and Brookshire, 1983; Trost, 1981), and is most often associated with neurologically based velopharyngeal incompetence (Trost, 1981). Both velar and palatal fricative are phonemic in some languages[111].

Psychological Problems

In addition to the many medical complication associated with orofacial clefts including feeding, hearing, and speech disorders, a variety of psychosocial difficulties occur at higher than eupected rates among children with clefts. These include externalizing and internalizing behaviour problems (Speltz et al[137], (1993); Richman[121], 1997); negative self evaluations (Kapp – Simon[74], 1986; and Mcguire, 1997); and learning disabilities, especially those related to reading and language (Richman, 1980; Richman et al[122], 1988; Broder et al[18], 1998).

Parent – Infant Bonding:

Several researchers and clinicians have also speculated that craniofacial conditions may have a detrimental effect on mother infant attachment (eg, Wadchter, 1997; Pillemer and Cook, 1989; Pruzansky, 1992; Rubin and Wilkinson, 1995). According to attachment theory, the bond between an infant and caregiver serves to protect the infant and ensure its survival (Bretherton[17], 1985). This function may be essentially important for babies who need extra care and attention, such as those with feeding problems and other medical challenges. Children with secure attachments are taught to develop confidence in others ability to care for them and belief in their own worthiness to receive such care. As they grow, these qualities help children negotiate the world successfully, even when caregivers are not physically present.

There are many obvious threats to parent –infant bonding, and they may not be as simple as was once assumed. Much of the research by Tobiasen (Tobiasen, 1984, 1987; Tobiasen and Heibert, 1993, 1993, 1994; Tobiasen et al[149]., 1987) focused on the adverse impact of abnormal facial appearance on early parent – child relationship as well as subsequent development of the child in the toddler, preschool, and school years. However, the research of Speltz and coworkers (Speltz, Armsden, and Clarren[139], 1990; Speltz, Galbreath, and Greeberg, 1995; Speltz et al., 1994) did not validate facial appearance as the predominant factor in parent – infant attachment.

Speltz et al[111] (1994) stated, "There is preliminary evidence for the existence of early difficulties in mother responsiveness and lack of clarity in the infant's communication of positive emotion and feeding cues. Such problems may lead to higher–than–average rates of insecure attachment, although this has yet to be investigated and should be a priority for future infancy research."

In contrast to previous theory and clinical speculation, the facial appearance of infants with CL/CP does not appear to affect the early mother infant relationship adversely. The infancy period is marked by attachment instability for infants with CP, who demonstrated lower than expected rates of security at 12 months. However, these problems resolved in nearly all cases by 24 months of age. Most infants with clefts emerged from the first 2 years of life with secure maternal attachments (Catherine L.Marie[26] (1999)).

Toddlers and Their Parents:

There are obvious conflicts in the data on toddlers with clefts (and other craniofacial anomalies) and their parents and in the conclusions that have been drawn. It is difficult to control all independent variables in any clinical investigation, and at this age there are rather " muddy" variables such as adequacy of previous surgical intervention in minimizing either facial disfigurement or speech defect, persistent ear disease despite myringotomies and tubes, and adjustment of parents to what can still be a self – perceived sense of inadequacy.

Pope[114] (1999) conjectured that ongoing medical attention gives the message (to the toddler) that he is not competent and that the world is too dangerous. However, she had no data verifying that medical interventions where frequent during the toddler period. She warned that carniofacial team members should be alert for signs of developmental and psychosocial disturbance in toddlers, a warning that is well taken.

The Preschool Years:

Obviously the areas of self–concept, behavior, and social skills are intricately tied together in children with craniofacial anomalies. The finding by Fisk et al[47] (1985) that "later" surgery in the 4- to 7- year age range produced more emotional problems coincides with the conclusion of Krueckeberg, Kapp-Simon, and Ribordy[77] (1993) that the preschool years may be a time relatively free of emotional stress. That is, the children in the study of Fisk et al (1985) evidenced greater emotional problems when their surgery stretched into the early school years as opposed to preschool.

Eliason[44] (1991) concluded that during the preschool years, a child's self-image and feelings about self are derived primarily from the parents' attitudes and behaviors. As the child's interaction with the world expands in the school years, the effects on self-image, socialization, school adjustment, and academic achievement become much more complex.

Intelligence, Learning Disabilities, School Achievement:

In their 1982 review of their own data and the published data of other authors on psychological characteristics of children with clefts, Richman and Eliason concluded the following with regard to school achievement:

(1) As a group, children with clefts tend to achieve below expectations based on their intellectual skills,

(2) Teachers tend to underestimate the intellectual ability of average and above – average children with more facial disfigurement,

(3) Children with clefts are frequently perceived as being more inhibited in the classroom,

(4) A general verbal or language deficiency in some children may result in ignificant academic failure, and

(5) Parents may have lower expectations for the cleft child, resulting in lower academic aspirations.

In their reviews, Mc Williams[93] (1982), Tobiasen[148] (1990) and Endriga and Kapp-Simon[75] (1999) emphasized many of these same points. Probably the most significant new finding with regard to school achievement that have emerged in recent years were those of Broder, Richman, and Mathewson[18] (1998), reviewed above. Certainly those findings brought to a halt any complacency clinicians had had that children with clefts were essentially normal by the time they reached the preadolescent or adolescent years.

Self Concept:

There are many factors potentially affecting self – concept and self – esteem in children with clefts and other craniofacial anomalies during the school – age year. Standardized tests and interviews tend to yield scores indicating lowered self – esteem, although this is not entirely consistent across studies and may be influenced by age, gender, severity of defect, parental attitudes, and so on. Pope (1999) made an excellent point to clinicians, namely, that it is important to be sensitive about what is communicated to the child about appearance because it will influence self – concept.

Personality, Behavior, Social Relationships:

Richman [121](1997) observed that the influence of cleft – related conditions on behavior at one age may not necessarily apply at another age for the same child and that many of the behavioral concerns may be transitory states amenable to change with intervention.

The data to date on psychosocial and educational concerns during the school – age years seem to indicate that children with clefts:

1. Are not apt to be significantly different from the peers in terms of personality measures or occurrence of psychopathology.
2. May be more apt to exhibit behavioral problems, with this difference to some extent dependent on age and gender.
3. May have some personality characteristics that differentiate them from noncleft peers, although the results seem to depend on sex, age, treatment success, and the particular independent variables chosen by investigators.
4. Are subject to teasing and other forms of abuse from peers and need assistance in learning how to handle this.
5. Are prone to difficulties in academic achievement, particularly in reading and other areas linked to language competencies.

A closer look at adolescents:

Endriga and Kapp-Simon[45] (1999) summarized the published information on psychosocial issues in teenagers with carniofacial anomalies. Global self – concept seems to fall within the normal range (Leonard et al., 1991; Starr, (1978). They stated that the literature indicated non-pathological elevations in inhibition and social introversion. Some subsets of teens (e.g. older adolescent girls) may be less well adjusted, perhaps owing to continued anxiety about facial appearance and its effect on social relationships. Adolescent girls do report more feelings of being unpopular, anxious, unhappy, and dissatisfied with their appearance (Broder, Smith, and Strauss[20], 1994; Kapp 1979; Leonary et al., 1991).

The work of Harper and Richman (1978) and Richman (1983) revealed dissatisfaction with educational and social functioning, self- doubt, and discomfort in interpersonal relationships. Tobiasen and Hiebert (1993) found that teens whose self –

ratings of facial impairment were less severe than peer ratings of that impairment had better self – esteem and psychosocial adjustment, as common sense would predict. Pope and Ward[114] (1997) found greater social competence in teenagers if the parents worried less about their child's friendships but at the same time actively encouraged the child's efforts to engage with peers.

Adults:

Clifford[30] (1979) concluded that individuals with clefts, as adults, assume reasonable positions in society and do not appear to be remarkably different from others. The data that have been derived in the intervening 20 years continue to support this conclusion. No consistent, significant differences between adults with clefts and control subjects have emerged in studies of educational levels, employment, or social integration.

Population based Scandinavian studies of young adults with facial clefts have shown that there is an impaired level of psychological well being among sub – groups of subjects with clefts (Ramsted et al, 1995). The risk of hospitalized mental disorders in general is increased in patients with CP but not to any substantial degree in patients with CL/CP. Both groups had an increased riks of mental retardation and substance abuse, but the risk for schizophrenia or bipolar illness was not statistically significantly increased, compared with the background population (Kaare Christesen[70], 2001).

ASSOCIATED MALFORMATIONS

Facial clefts are often associated with other anomalies or syndromes (Cohen[33] 1991). The reported frequency of associated anomalies and syndromes varies widely depending on the definition of associated anomalies and the time and extent of follow-up. However, a consistent finding is the higher frequency of associated anomalies and syndromes among patients with isolated cleft palate (CP; usually in the range of 13% to 50%) than among patients with cleft lip with or without cleft palate (CL / CP) cases (typically in the range of 2% to 13%; Gorlin et al, 1990).

Syndromes and congenital malformations by organ system (C Stoll[141] 2000,)
Table.7.1

Chromosmoe Syndromes	Digestive system
Trisomy 13	Esophageal atresia
Trisomy 18	Deodenal atresia
del (4q)	Diverticule of meckel
del (2q)	Anal atresia
del (13q)	Common mesenter
	Other
Partal autesomal trisomes (1q, 9p, 10p)	**Respiratory system**
47, XXX	Choanal atresia

47 XXY	Nose anomalies
45, X	Laryngeal anomalies
46 Xr(X)	Pulmonary agenesia
45, X/ 46, XY	Other
45, X/ 47, XXX	
Recognized non chromosomal syndrome	**Ear**
Cornelia de Lange syndrome	Auricular malformation and deafness
Ivemark	Auricular malformation
Multiple pterygium	**Facial anomalies**
Velo – cardio – facial	**Skeletal anomalies**
Oro – facio – digital	
Klippel – feil	Club foot
VATER	Club hand
Moebius	Polydactyly
Stickler	Syndactyly
Otopalato digital	Limb deficiency -upper limb
Goldenhar	Limb deficiency -lower limb
Meckel	Limb deficiency -both limb
Adams – oliver	**Cardiovascular system**
Treacher – Collins	Ventricular septal defect
Omen reticulo endotheliose	Auricular septal defect
Congenital anomalies by organ system (syndromes excluded)	Tetralogy of fallot
Central nervous system	Atrioventricular canal
Anencephaly	Pulmonary stenosis
Spinabifida	Coarctation of aorta
Encephalocele	**The eye**
Microcephaly	Anopthalmia
Agenesia corpus collosum	Micropthalmia
Hydrocephaly	Bupthalmia
	Cataracte
	Coloboma
Urogenital	**Abdominal wall**
Renal agenesia bilateral	Diaphragmatic hernia
Renal agenesia unilateral	Omphalocele
Hydronephrosis	**Skin**
Ureteral anomalies	Scalp agenesia
Megaureter	Other
Horse shoe kidney	
Vesical exstrophy	
Vesicoureteral reflex	
Hypospodias	

Chapter-8

MULTIDISCIPLINARY APROACH IN MANAGEMENT OF CLEFT LIP AND PALATE

The American Academy of Pediatric Dentistry, in its efforts to promote optimal health for children with cleft lip/palate and other craniofacial anomalies endorses the following current statements of the American Cleft – Palate – Craniofacial Association[3].

Fundamental Principles:
Several fundamental principles were identified as critical to optimal cleft/craniofacial care. These principles are:

1. Management of patients with craniofacial anomalies is best provided by an interdisciplinary team of specialists.

2. Optimal care for patients with craniofacial anomalies is provided by teams that see sufficient numbers of these patients each year to maintain clinical expertise in diagnosis and treatment.

3. Although referral for team evaluation and management is appropriate for patients of any age, the optimal time for the first evaluation is within the first few weeks of life and, whenever possible, within the first few days.

4. From the time of first contact with the child and family, every effort must be made to assist the family in adjusting to the birth of a child with a craniofacial anomaly and to the consequent demands and stress placed upon that family.

5. Parents/caregivers must be given information about recommended treatment procedures, options, risk factors, benefits, and costs to assist them in   a) making informed decisions on the child's behalf, and b) preparing the child and themselves for all recommended procedures.   The team should actively solicit family participation and collaboration in treatment planning and, when the child is mature enough to do so, he or she should also participate in treatment decisions.

6. Treatment plans should be developed and implemented on the basis of team recommendations.

7. Care should be coordinated by the team, but should be provided at the local level whenever possible; however, complex diagnostic or surgical procedures should be restricted to major centers with appropriate treatment facilities and experienced care providers.

8. It is the responsibility of each team to be sensitive to linguistic, cultural, ethnic, psychosocial, economic, and physical factors that affect the dynamic relationship between the team and the patient and family.

9. It is the responsibility of the team to monitor both short term and long- term outcomes. Thus, longitudinal follow up of patients, including appropriate documentation and record keeping, is essential.

10. Evaluation of treatment outcomes must take into account the satisfaction and psychosocial well being of the patient as well as effects on growth, function and appearance.

Treatment planning and protocols

A step by step analysis involving first a history, then examination, both clinical and by special investigations, followed by a diagnosis, is the classical approach to treatment planning in most clinical situations. Unfortunately such a system has little application to the very complex and varied problems that present in the congenital deformity of ceft lip and palate. There is no single protocol to be applied universally several medical centers are following their own treatment plan and protocols for treating their cleft lip and palate patients.

Table –8.1.**Protocol recommended by A Cameron and R.Widmer[2] (1997)**

Age	Paedodontic	Orthodontic	General Practitioner	Surgical
Birth	Initial contact and interview with parents. Registration with cleft palate scheme. Arrange contact with parental support groups.	Construction of presurgical orthopaedic appliance if required.		Initial assessment.
3-5 months	Initial contact, if not at birth. Introduce dental care plan. Study models at time of lip repair.			Primary surgical repair of lip.
12 months	Review			Surgical repair of palate.
2-6 years	12 monthly reviews for assessment of growth and development, caries and preventive advice.		Initial visit, then 6 monthly for preventive advice, topical fluoride applicationand fissure sealing.	Possible revision of lip repair. Pharyngoplasty if required. Myringotomy and grommets by ENT.
6-7 years	Fissure sealing of first		Fissure sealing	Myringotomy

	permanent molars. Composite resin restoration of hypoplastic teeth adjacent to cleft. Preventive advice.		of first permanent molars. Composite resin restoration of hypoplastic teeth adjacent to cleft. Preventive advice.	and grommets by ENT as required.
8-10 year	Case conference with surgical and orthodontic teams for bone grafting.	Assessment for maxillary expansion prior to bone grafting. Skeletal age assessments.	6 - monthly reviews. Possible extractions of erupted supernume-rary teeth. Interim bridge or partial denture.	Bone grafting at one- half to two thirds root development of canine.
11-12 years	Retention of palatal expansion.		6 – monthly reviews	
12-15 years	12 monthly review	Full fixed appliance therapy.	Fissure – sealing of bicuspids and second molars.	Review and possible surgical revision if required.
16-17 years	Restoration of teeth adjacent to cleft. Referral to general practitioner.	Retention post orthodontic therapy.	Restoration of teeth in the cleft, including crowns, bridges, implants & dentures.	Assessment of the need for orthognathic surgery.

Table- 8.2.Treatment scheme provided by AHR Rowe et al[4] (1995)

Age	Plastic surgery	Oral surgery	Orthodontics	Speech therapy	ENT
Birth	Assessment of problem and discussion with parents		Full records from birth to maturity. Presurgical orthopaedics in		

			some cases.		
3 months 1-1 ½ years	Lip repair Palate repair				Regular monitoring from 1st year to adulthood.
2 ½ years				Assessme-nt of speech at 2½ years, but reas-surance and observation before hand	
4-5	Revision of lip or palate				
5 + years	Surgery for speech defects				
8-9 years			Simple orthodontic treatment to correct incisor crossbites and / or facilitate alveolar bone grafting	Speech therapy when required	
10 years		Alveolar bone grafting			
12-14 years			Definitive orthodontic treatment		
16 years	Revision of nose				
17-18 years		Major maxillary surgery if maxillary hypoplasia, and orthognathic surgery to correct jaw deformities.	Bridge and denture work.		

There appear to be as many variations in technique, sequencing and timing of treatment as there are cleft palate teams. There are, however, some commonly accepted aims and principles of treatment.

Aims of Cleft Treatment:

The ultimate goal is to attain normal form and function (especially speech and mastication) with the least possible damage to growth and development through surgical intervention.

Specific treatment objectives are:

1.   Provide a long mobile palate capable of completely closing off the oropharynx from the nasopharynx.

2.   Produce a full upper lip with a symmetrical Cupid's bow and reconstruction of the columella and the alar architecture of the nose.

3.   Achieve an intact, well-aligned dental arch with a stable inter-arch occlusion.

Dental Care (recommended by American Academy of Pediatric Dentistry[3] in 2000):

As members of the interdisciplinary team of physicians, dentists, speech pathologists, and other allied health professionals, paediatric dentists should provide dental services in close cooperation with their orthodontic, oral and maxillofacial surgery, and prosthodontic colleagues. All dental specialists should ensure that:

1. Dental radiographs, cephalometric radiographs, and other imaging modalities as indicated should be utilized to evaluate and monitor dental and facial growth and development.

2. Diagnostic records, including properly occluded dental study models, should be collected at appropriate intervals for patients at risk for developing malocclusion or maxillary- mandibular discrepancies.

3. Presurgical maxillary orthopedics to improve the position of the maxillary alveolar segments prior to surgical closure of the lip may be indicated for some infants.

4. As the primary dentition erupts, the team evaluation should include a dental examination and, if such services are not already being provided, referral to appropriate providers for caries control, preventive measures, and space management.

5. Before the primary dentition has completed eruption, the skeletal and dental components should be evaluated to determine if a malocclusion is present or developing.

6. Depending upon the specific goals to be accomplished and also upon the age at which the patient is initially evaluated, orthodontic management of the malocclusion may be performed in the primary, mixed, or permanent dentition. In some cases, orthodontic treatment may be necessary in all three stages.

7. While continuous active orthodontic treatment from early mixed dentition to permanent dentition should be avoided, each stage of orthodontic therapy may be followed by retention and regular observation. Orthodontic retention for the permanent dentition may extend into adulthood.

8. For some patients with craniofacial anomalies, functional orthodontic appliances may be indicated.

9. For patients with craniofacial anomalies, orthodontic treatment may be needed in conjunction with surgical correction of the facial deformity.

10. Congenitally missing teeth may be replaced with a removable appliance, fixed restorative bridgework, or osseointegrated implants.

11.Patients should be closely monitored for dental and periodontal disease.

12.Prosthetic obturation of palatal fistulae may be necessary in some patients.

13. Aprosthetic speech device may be used to treat velopharyngeal inadequacy in some patients.

The Cleft Palate Team

The cleft palate team may be defined as a team of professionals who provide coordinated and interdisciplinary evaluation and treatment to patients with CL/CP.

Whitehouse has described the clinical team as a "close, cooperative, democratic, multi-professional union devoted to a common purpose – the best treatment of the fundamental needs of the patient"[147].

The Cleft palate team comprises:
1. Plastic surgeons
2. Pediatric dentists
3. Paediatrician
4. Orthodontists
5. Speech pathologists

6. Oral maxillofacial surgeons
7. Ear, nose and throat surgeons/ Otolaryngologist
8. Social workers
9. Nurses/ Dietician
10. Psychologists
11. Other specialists, such as geneticists, who are consulted as required in individual cases

A Cleft palate team should meet face to face for regularly scheduled meetings for treatment planning and case review, with a minimum of six meeting times per year. The interaction between disciplines is likely to result in improved treatment plans and more coordination between providers.

For patients requiring orthognathic treatment the cleft palate team would have an orthodontist well prepared for the provision of a orthognatic treatment. All orthognathic surgical treatment should be documented with preoperative and postoperative dental study models, facial and intraoral radiographs and cephalometric radiographs. In all cases of persons with cleft lip and palate, orthognathic surgical planning and outcomes should be routinely discussed at the cleft palate team meetings.

The paediatric dentists and prosthodontist may serve to evaluate and treat dental conditions associated with cleft.

Cleft palate team should have a speech language pathologist who attends team meetings and who is educated and equipped to diagnose and treat patients with cleft lip and palate. On a cleft palate team, the speech language pathologist routinely performs a structured speech assessment during team evaluations and uses clinical speech instrumentation (such as endoscopy, pressure flow, video fluoroscopy, etc) to assess velopharyngeal function when indicated.

Consultation from otolaryngologist should be undertaken when a hearing loss is detected. Hearing evaluation routinely includes a test by an audiologist and an ear examination by an otolaryngologist before 1 year of age.

The psychological and social issues related to facial clefting suggest that the team have a psychologist, clinical social worker or other mental health professional who evaluates all patients on a regular basis. Furthermore the team should routinely test or screen patients for learning disabilities and developmental, psychological, and language skills.

The team should use a nurse or other trained professional who regularly provides supportive counseling and instruction (feeding and developmental) to interested parents of newborns.

The involvement of primary care physicians on the team (paediatrician, family physician, or general internist) may be of great importance in detecting and responding to health problems of team patients. The regular attendance at team meetings of a primary care physician also assists in linking to community providers.

The cleft palate team should also provide formal genetic counseling or a clinical genetic evaluation for patients or patients who desire such evaluation.

All cleft palate team should keep a central and shared file on each patients. The clinical files or records of the cleft palate team should routinely include:

1. One or more diagnoses
2. A complete medical history
3. A treatment plan or goals that are reviewed periodically
4. A social and psychological history
5. Dental and orthodontic findings and history
6. Intraoral dental casts of patients, when indicated
7. Facial photographs of patients in treatment or evaluation
8. Lateral cephalometric radiographs of patients when indicated

After a cleft palate team evaluation, the patient and family should routinely have an opportunity to ask questions and discuss the treatment plan with a team representative. Further more, the team routinely should write reports, summary letters, containing a treatment plan, to the family. The cleft palate team routinely provides case management and benefits advocacy / assistance, as needed. In order to function, it should have an office and coordinator or secretary.

Initial consultation:

1. Examination of the baby:
The baby is examined and a record made of the type of cleft or other deformity present and the relation of the lip, alveolar and palatal clefts (i.e. arch form etc.), with a note of any overriding of segments, distortion of premaxilla, etc. Any erupted teeth are charted and a note made of any natal or neonatal teeth in the cleft or other regions.

Medical history:
A full medical history must be conducted at this time. Many clefts are merely one component in one of the 50 clefting syndromes and it is common for other congenital abnormalities to be present in addition to the cleft (e.g. congenital heart disease).

Dental records:
1. Photographs should be taken at all major review visits.
2. Dental impressions should be taken by the paediatric dentist, or the plastic surgeon under general anaesthesia before the lip repair.

3. An initial screening panoramic radiography is useful at 5-6 years of age (or earlier if pathology is present or suspected).
4. All Children should have study models and panoramic dental radiographs and lateral cephalometric radiographs at 8-9 years of age.

The parental interview about dental care:

If the parents are not present when the baby is examined, a separate appointment must be made with them. The parent interview is one of the most important aspects of the initial consultation.

The approach in speaking to parents at this consultation should be relaxed and informative–a mostly 'getting to know you' introduction of the dental team as a preparation for later visits. It must be remembered that because of the emotional impact of the facial abnormality on the mother, father and family, they may not be fully receptive to advice at this early visit or remember much of what is said. At this interview it is important to explain.

➢   The dental aspects of the clefting process.

➢   The likely course of dental management. The involvement of different specialities, including restorative, radiological, orthodontic, and possible later oral surgical care.

➢   The probability of the absence of the normal tooth in the region of the cleft and the presence of one or more supernumerary teeth instead in the cleft region should be mentioned.

➢   The likelihood of the presence of crown and root morphological abnormalities and enamel hypoplasia of the incisor and canine teeth adjacent to the cleft should be indicated with the positive reassurance that these can be treated relatively simply soon after they appear.

➢   The absolute importance of sound preventive care and regular dental visit should be emphasized.

It will almost certainly be necessary to reinforce the introductory information and advice given at this visit at many subsequent outpatient visits over the years of treatment. Many cleft palate clinics produce parent handbooks, which are particularly useful.

Role of the Paediatric Dentist

The role of the paediatric dentist is one of coordinator. Between the ages of 12 and 18 months the paediatric dentist should see the child at regular intervals no greater than 12 months. In some countries the child is enrolled in the Cleft Palate

Scheme at the first visit. This scheme provides government health benefits to pay for orthodontic, surgical and some general dental treatment. Parental support groups such as Cleft Pals are present in many countries and contact should be arranged as soon as possible with these organizations.

First Follow – up Visit:

> Dental charting is carried out, including a record of the time of eruption of first tooth.

> Body growth should be checked and height/ weight entered on a growth chart. Details can be obtained from the child's Health Record Book.

These visits are essential for the general monitoring of growth and development and the control of dental disease. Updating of photographic, study model and radiological records will also be done. The paediatric dentist will generally coordinate all dental care aspects with those of other disciplines.

Preventive Dental Care:

Preventive dental care is essential for these patients using all known techniques including:

> Tooth brushing.
> Home self – application of topical fluoride.
> Fissure sealing of both primary and permanent teeth.
> Oral hygiene technique instruction.
> Dietary advice to child and parents by paediatric dentist (or dietitian if necessary)

The prevention of dental carries and periodontal disease will help with cooperation for ultimate definitive orthodontic treatment by reducing unpleasant visits for treatment in early childhood. Motivation is especially important for later orthodontic treatment in these patients. This should be assessed early, and enhanced during preventive visits during childhood[2].

General dental practitioner care

The role of the general dental practitioner is paramount. Child with craniofacial anomalies has significantly greater rates of dental disease, all of which is preventable and will affect the prognosis and course of future treatment. The child should if possible attend a general dental practitioner at 6 monthly intervals for preventive care, dietary advice and oral hygiene technique follow-up, together with routine restorative care if necessary. The parents should agree to attend the local dentist regularly. One of the most important duties is to establish early contact with the cleft palate team or surgeon and maintain a frequent dialogue.

Dental Extractions and Minor Oral Surgery:

1.   Except in an emergency, the general dentist should not do dental extractions for these children without first checking and clearing this with the supervising paediatric dentist or orthodontist.
2.   Primary molars should be retained by pulpotomy, or the space maintained after extraction as advised by the paediatric dentist.
3.   Erupted supernumerary teeth should be retained until 6 to 7 years of age, unless impossible to clean, resulting in progressive dental caries, gingival or mucosal inflammation.

Extraction of such teeth should then, in most cases, be carried out in the supervising hospital either under local or general anaesthesia. If general anaesthesia is required superficial or obstructing unerupted supernumerary teeth may be removed at the same time, but only after discussion with the coordinating paediatric dentist. If a bone graft is planned for the alveolar cleft, the paediatric dentist coordinator may advise retaining unerupted supernumerary teeth especially if it is one of the permanent tooth series. The maxillofacial surgeon removes this tooth at the time of bone grafting.

Role of Orthodontist

With in the cleft palate team the orthodontist is the one dentist most likely to see a cleft patient right through from birth to maturity; and certainly in the younger patient, he must not only carry out any necessary treatment of a specialist nature, but also act as a coordinator for all other types of dental treatment. For example, orthodontit must ensure that satisfactory general dental care is available for the child at the appropriate age.

Orthodontic treatment can take place at various stages of development from birth to maturity, but to avoid overtaxing the patient's power of cooperation it is wise to concentrate appliance therapy into limited periods of continuous active treatment, with the main emphasis on the permanent dentition.

I. In the new born period (birth to 3 or 5 months)

In cases of bilateral cleft lip and palate, the infant has a premaxillary segment that is either positioned severely anterior to the maxillary arch segments or deviated laterally to one side of the cleft defect. In this case, if the lip surgeries under taken without presurgical orthodontic correction, there is more chances of lip dehiscence.

Presurgical Orthopedics:

The goal of presurgical orthopedics in unilateral clefts of the lip and palate is to bring the cleft segment into alignment with the noncleft side to minimize the width of the defect. In bilateral clefts the goals are (1) to bring the unattached premaxilla into better alignment with both of the lateral alveolar segments and (2) to keep the lateral segments from moving inward behind the premaxilla both before and after lip surgery.

1) The Premaxillary Retractor Appliance:

As early as 1686, Hofman described the use of a head cap and premaxillary strap to reposition the premaxilla. This type of apparatus is useful in anteroposterior and vertical repositioning.

The premaxillary retraction appliance is constructed and inserted after 1 week of insertion of intra oral obturator into cleft palate. This intra oral obturator is constructed as soon as possible after birth of child having cleft palate defect. After delivery of obturator, the infant is allowed to become accustomed to the appliance for a 1 week period. At the second appointment the infant is fitted with a premaxillary retraction appliance.

Technique:

A baby bonnet is made to provide "headgear" anchorage for a premaxillary retraction strap. An elastic strap is placed over the protracting premaxilla and anchored to the infant head with the bonnet (fig. 8.1). By the application of sequentially increasing equal forces to the premaxilla, the premaxilla is retropositioned into a more normal position relative to the maxillary segments. This bonnet and strap appliance is worn 24 hours a day and is removed only for feeding. The desired movement can usually be accomplished within 6 to 8 weeks.

In a laterally deviated premaxilla in an infant with a bilateral cleft lip and palate, this appliance would not place the premaxilla in the facial midline. Therefore the premaxilla must be positioned in the midline before premaxillary retraction.

In this clinical presentation, an impression is made of the infant's premaxilla for construction of external acrylic "bulb" prosthesis. This appliance is fitted over the protruding and laterally displaced premaxilla and anchored to the infant's head with a bonnet appliance. By application of sequentially increasing differential forces, the premaxilla is brought into the facial midline.

The rationale for use of a bulb prosthesis before elastic strap retraction includes the following consideration:
1. The bulb prosthesis affords greater control over the differential forces applied to the premaxilla.
2. Movement of the premaxilla into the facial midline before retropositioning decreases the risk of distorting a vomer stalk.
3. The consideration of a surgical premaxillary setback is eliminated.
4. Optimal premaxillary positioning may eliminate the need for a staged lip closure, thereby decreasing total hospitalization time and cost.
5. The appearance of the nose and lip is improved by the fact that the lip incisions can be surgically closed under less tension and by an underlying symmetric alignment of the alveolar segments.

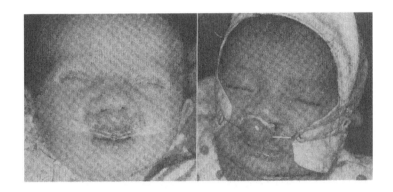

Fig.8.1 Baby bonnet

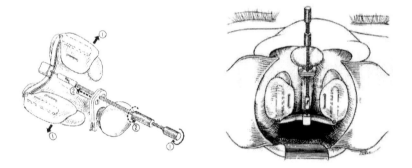

Fig.8.2 Pin retained appliance

2) The Expansion Appliances:

The construction of expansion prosthesis for infants with bilateral cleft lip and palate was recommended by McNeil[90] (1954), Burston[24] (1958) and Harkins 60 (1960). As described by Harkins, the sequence of treatment when expansion prosthesis is used is as follows;

1. Initial and secondary impressions.
2. Construction of the expansion prosthesis.
3. Resection of the vomer (now soldom done).
4. Placement of the expansion prosthesis in site.
5. Surgical closure of the lip.
6. Surgical closure of the alveolar process after retroposition of the premaxillary process.
7. Surgical (or prosthetic) restoration of the palate at a later age.

The appliance will not only act as a retainer and prevent maxillary collapse but also stimulate growth. The appliance also alleviates the feeding problem and has a beneficial effect on future speech function.

Early orthodontic therapy without surgical interference was reported by McNeil in 1956 [89]. He used a palatal appliance to keep the palatal segments apart before the palate was repaired. He believed that constriction of the maxilla could not be avoided after lip surgery. Therefore he recommended repositioning of the parts before lip surgery, he maintained that his series of split palatal appliances contributed toward bone growth and resulted in narrowing of the hard palate cleft. The splints are constructed at specific age intervals and are split in the midline and periodically realigned to move the palatal segments into a more normal anatomic relation. After orthodontic repositioning, the cleft lip and nose are surgically repaired, and a gingivoplasty is frequently accomplished.

The Pin-retained Appliance:

Georgiade [56](1971) and Latham[78], kusy, and Georgiade (1976) proposed the use of pin-retained appliances to expand the collapsed alveolar segments while retracting the premaxilla in the bilateral Cleft. This was followed by lip closure and gingivoplasty where possible (fig.8.2).

Lathams Appliance:

Latham (1980) described a pin-retained appliance used to advance the cleft maxillary alveolar segment in the unilateral cleft cases. The goal is to correct the retropositioned alveolar process and in so doing, improve support for the alar base on the cleft side. After initial lip and nasal repair and gingivoplasty, the palate is expanded with a fixed, pin-retained appliance and held in place for retention (one to two months). The principle is to correct the reduction in arch circumference that was associated with orthopedic activity before the adoption of gingival, labial, and nasal surgical repair. The goal of postsurgical orthopedic expantion and retention is to overcorrect the postsurgically reduced arch width. No bone grafting is done in these procedures.

Before closure of the gingival tissue, the periodontium is teased toward the opposite cleft wall in order to encourage primary bone deposition. The pre-and postsurgical orthopedic control of the unilateral cleft palate, as described above, produces an arch that is usually resistant to medial collapse.

The presurgical infant orthopedics, when combined with gingivoperiosteoplasty (GPP), eliminates the need for alveolar bone grafting in the mixed dentition period. Gingivoperiosteoplasty is the primary repair of the gingivoperiosteum at the site of alveolar cleft, with the intention of forming an osseous union. This approach has recently advocated by Millard and Latham[97] (1990). This new method is quite different from the surgical approach of Skoog[137] (1965) in which preoperative orthopedics was not used and wide subperiosteal undermining was employed with presurgical orthopedics. Gingivoperiosteal repair can be performed with minimal undermining and with a narrow bone gap that must be bridged.

Previously all children with complete alveolar clefts were likely to require alveolar bone graft during the period of mixed dentition. Narrowing of the alveolar cleft and approximating the lateral segments through presurgical infant orthopedics followed by GPP at the time of lip repair may eliminate the need for this bone graft (Pedro E. Santigo[108] 1998).

It is generally accepted that, in the absence of postsurgical overexpansion, the retention forces exerted by the repaired lip musculature may displace one or both of the maxillary segments medially (Pruzansky and Aduss, [116]1967). It is also an established fact that early orthodontic treatment can effectively reposition the malposed segments. As a result, not only are the maldeveloped and displaced segments positioned more anatomically but the existing crossbite malocclusion is also corrected (Subtelny and Brodie, 1954; Subtelny, 1966; Coccano[32], 1970).

3) Presurgical Nasoalveolar Moulding

Presurgical nasoalveloar moulding (PNAM) is a new approach to the traditional method of presurgical infant orthopedics for patients with unilateral and bilateral clefts of the lip, alveolus, and palate. The PNAM treatment protocol for patients has been described by Grayson et al[58].(1993), Brecht et al[16].(1995), Graysons and Santiago (1997), and Cutting et al[37].(1998). This treatment modality includes as its objectives the active moulding and repositioning of the deformed nasal cartilages and alveolar processes, as well as the lengthening of the deficient columella.

METHODS

Correction of the *Unilateral* Oronasal Cleft Deformity:

The goals of PNAM in the unilateral CL/CP patient are to align and approximate the introral alveolar segments and to correct the malposition of the nasal cartilages. In addition, the nasal tip and the alar base on the affected side, as well as the position of the philtrum and columella, are corrected (Bardach and Cutting[9], 1990). These corrections are achieved using an acrylic intraoral moulding plate with a nasal stent rising from the labial vestibular flange(8.3).

At one to two weeks after birth, members of the interdisciplinary cleft palate team evaluate the infant. Following the clinical examination, an impression of the intraoral cleft defect is made using an elastomeric material in an infant acrylic impression tray.

An impression of the nasal region may be helpful for comparision of the pre and post nasoalvoelar moulding results or to aid in the fabrication of a nasal stent. A conventional moulding plate is fabricated on the maxillary cast using clear acrylic resin.
The moulding plate is secured to the palate and alveolar processes through the use of surgical adhesive tape that are applied externally to the cheeks and to an acrylic extension from the oral plate that is positioned between the lips under the cleft.

The moulding plate is modified at weekly intervals to gradually approximate the alveolar segments and to reduce the size of the intraoral cleft gap.
The Nasal Stent:

When the alveolar cleft width has been reduced to less than 6mm, the nasal stent may be added to the moulding plate appliance so that nasal cartilage moulding may begin.

The nasal stent is a projection of acrylic that is fabricated on the labial flange of the oral moulding plate. Through gradual additions of small amounts of acrylic resin, the stent is positioned inside the nose underneath the apex of the alar cartilage on the cleft side. The alar dome cartilage on the cleft side is lifted by the stent to achieve normal elevation and symmetry. The base of the stent should be located midway between the cleft lip segments. At the active tip of the nasal stent, the acrylic is covered with a thin veneer of soft denture lining material to insure that tissue breakdown do not happen when positive pressure is applied to the nasal lining. The stent serves as a custom tissue expander for the cleft side of the columella. The elevation of the nasal tip on the cleft side will also increase the patency of the nostril aperture.

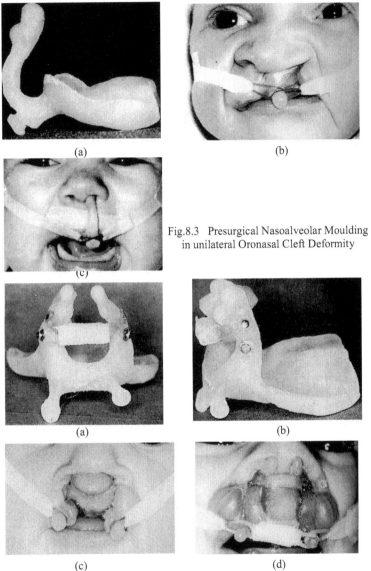

(a)   (b)

Fig.8.3   Presurgical Nasoalveolar Moulding
in unilateral Oronasal Cleft Deformity

(c)

(a)   (b)

(c)   (d)
Fig. 8.4 Presurgical Nasoalveolar Moulding in bilateral Oronasal Cleft Deformity

Through gradual modifications made weekly to the nasal stent, the shape of the cartilaginous septum, alar cartilage tip, and medial and lateral crus are carefully molded to resemble the normal shape of these structures.

Correcting the *Bilateral* Oronasal Cleft Defromity

The objectives of PNAM in the bilateral CL/CP patient are to lengthen the columella, to reposition the apex of the alar cartilages toward the tip, and to align the alveolar segments and premaxilla to form a normal maxillary arch.

After completion of the initial clinical evaluation by members of the cleft palate team, an impression of the intraoral and nasal cleft defect is obtained in a manner similar to that described previously for the unilateral cleft defect. An intraoral moulding plate is fabricated that encompasses the lateral alveolar segments and the premaxilla. The first stage of treatment includes repositioning of the everted premaxilla into the space between the lateral alveolar segments, which is accomplished through progressive modification of the acrylic intraoral moulding plate, as previously described. A combination of elastic bands and surgical tape is adhered to the cheeks or attached to a head cap to actively position the moulding plate against the premaxilla and alveolar segments (fig.8.4).

In the second stage (after approximately three weeks of treatment), a pair of nasal stent is built up from the anterior flange of the oral moulding plate to enter the nasal apertures. The nasal stents elevate the nasal cartilages and provide resistance to downward pull by tape placed on the prolabium. A horizontal prolabial band pulls back on the base of the columella at the nasolabial fold; the band's force is directed to preserve the nasolabial angle at the junction of the columella base and philtrum as the columella is lengthened.

Complications of Nasoalveolar Moulding:

1.   Soft tissue breakdown may occur when modifications of the appliance are excessive, resulting in force application that exceeds tissue tolerance. An area of ulceration may develop intraoarlly or on the nasal lining where active moulding pressure is applied.

2.   If parents fail to properly apply tape and elastics during moulding, then the appliance will not be adequately retained during the course of treatment, the progress will be lost.

Advantages Provided by PNAM:

Recent clinical studies support the role of nasoalveolar moulding in correcting the nasal cartilage deformity, columella length deficiency, and alveolar malposition prior to the primary surgical repiar (Maull et al.,[88]1997; Wood et al.,[165]1997).

1. Pre-Surgical reduction of the alveolar cleft gap enables the surgeon to perform a gingivoperiosteoplasty. This procedure has been shown to reduce the need for secondary alveolar bone grafting during the period of the mixed dentition in more than 60% of the case studies (Santiago et al., [133]1998) and thus far does not appear to adversely affect facial growth (Wood et al., [165]1997).

2. The presurgical alignment and correction of the deformity in the nasal cartilages minimizes the extent of the primary nasal surgery required, thereby also minimizing the formation of scar tissue and producing more consistent postoperative results.

3. In the bilateral cleft deformity, nonsurgical columella lengthening eliminates the need for secondary surgical columella elongation and the accompanying scars at the lip-columella junction.

4. PNAM, when used in conjunction with a modified surgical approach, allows for a single initial surgical procedure to address the lip-nose- alveolus complex and its deformity, thereby reducing the number and extent of surgeries that a cleft patient will undrgo during a lifetime (Cutting et al., 1998).

II. Period of Deciduous Dentition:

Treatment during this phase of dental development is initially focused on establishing and maintaining optimal oral health i.e. keeping the teeth healthy, preventing baby bottle caries, seeing to it that restorations are carried out when necessary, and intervening to prevent ill-advised dental extractions.

Little orthodontic intervention is required during this stage, although contact is maintained with the family to ensure that the general dental health is satisfactory and, that once the deciduous dentition is becoming established, the child is registered with a local dental practitioner.

Meticulous daily oral hygiene for the child, emphasizing direct assistance from the parents, is established to reduce the possibility of developing dental decay. Special care should be taken to keep the ectopically erupted teeth free from decay because food often becomes lodged in and around the cleft defect.

An increase in periodic recall examinations possibly at 3 to 4 months intervals enables the dentist to intercept areas of decay. This preventive regimen is continued throughout all subsequent stages in the management of the cleft patient.

Orthodontic management in this period:

i)   In some extensive cases of unilateral and bilateral complete clefts of the lips and palate, surgical closure of the palatal defect is postponed beyond the usual 18 to 24 months of age. In these cases, because of the development of speech at this age, maxillary prosthetic appliances are constructed to provide normal maxillary arch integrity. As the child grows, more tissue will become available to close the palate when doing so is surgically appropriate.

2.   Early orthodontic correction in the child with a congenital cleft lip and palate has been recommended by many U.S. orthodontists and is initiated after the eruption of all deciduous teeth. When the child is approximately 3 ½ years of age.

The advantages of early treatment are many particularly in the areas of function, esthetics and speech. In addition, a foundation is provided for the support of the surgically reconstructed lip. The dentition must be in satisfactory condition, not only to permit the use of fixed orthodontic appliances but also to allow prolonged use of retention appliances. The repositioning of the displaced palatal segments of the maxilla is dependent on the presence of teeth, both deciduous and permanent. Since teeth serve to support the orthodontic appliance, dental care of the deciduous teeth is imperative and specialists in paediatric dentistry must be consulted.

Early orthodontic intervention is indicated in children showing sign of malocclusion such as incisor, or buccal segment crossbite and in some bilateral cleft cases, protrusion of the premaxillary segment. Unfortunately, corrections of these defects will not remain stable and therefore continuous retention will be required.

3.   In some bilateral clefts in which the lateral palatal segments are locked behind premaxillary segment, an advancement of premaxilla is indicated before an attempt is made to move constricted palatal segments laterally.

Vargervik [160] (1990 & 1995) suggested that orthodontic treatment may begin during this period, however, if there is a significant collapse of the maxillary segment on the side of the cleft and particularly if the mandible shifts into an occlusal relationship with the collapsed segment. If such a situation is left untreated, the functional shift of the mandible may lead to a permanent unfavorable position of the lower jaw even – after the permanent dentition erupts.

For the most part, however, orthodontic therapy is not undertaken in the deciduous dentition phase because the effects are unlikely to be sustained in the permanent dentition (Asher–McDade and Sham[160], 1990).

Pruzansky and Aduss, [116]1967; Coccano[32] 1970 have found a high percentage of orthodontic collapse as represented by a crossbite in the deciduous dentition. Collapse of maxillary arch is a factor in many cleft palate patients, and it was shown to occur in 40 percent of all cases in one study.

Moore [101](1986) pointed out that the need for long – term retention (long term use of appliances to keep the teeth in the desired position) could, in the deciduous dentition, actually impede growth.

III. Period of Mixed Dentition:

In this period, there may be several areas of concern for the orthodontist when the permanent first molar and incisors erupt. The most commonly recurring features are incisor and buccal segment crossbites, malalignments (especially in the region of the cleft), some constriction of maxillary arch form, missing permanent teeth (notably the upper lateral incisors), and abnormal paths of mandibular closure.

Orthodontic management in this period:

1. Individual tooth derotation and arch alignment can be accomplished by orthodontic fixed appliance therapy. It is often impossible to attain a correct midline relationship, a fairly consistent problem.
2. Correction of class III incisor relationship may be possible at this stage. If this cross bite is due to dentoalveolar discrepancy, it can be corrected by an acrylic inclined plane secured to the mondibular incisors. (Proclination of upper incisors has a more favourable prognosis in bilateral cleft cases since here the maxillary dental base is often slightly protrusive and the incisor crossbite is due to the lingual rotation of the premaxillary segment and retroclination of upper incisors)
3. Misplaced teeth or supernumerary teeth, over retained deciduous teeth that have erupted in the line of cleft, can be removed without any disadvantages, especially if they become carious or create a stagnation area that is difficult to clean.
4. Vargervik, 1995, has advised to do the expansion of the maxilla and straightening of the incisors. It can be accomplished with a lingual appliance, sometimes, with a spring that gives more of a push to the anterior part of the lateral maxillary segment than the posterior part (fig.8.5). It can be kept for retention purpose in the late mixed dentition stage.
5. In the age range of 9 to 12 years, the orthodontist will be focusing on correction of maxillary width in preparation for alveolar bone grafting. If maxillary expansion and protraction was began earlier, that treatment can continue while the remaining permanent teeth erupt. Face mask may be used in the effort to bring the maxilla forward (fig.8.6). Some of the fixed appliances are used for maxillary expansion and correction of the position of individual teeth.
6. It appears that a rapid palatal expansion bite-plane appliance offers the orthodontist the ability to effectively treat patient with maxillary arch width deficiency. While the appliance does not have acrylic palatal contact to assist in recontouring the palate, it does effectively permit maxillary expansion and protraction. It is also possible that bite planes may lessen root resorption and TMJ microtrauma by removing interfering heavy biting forces, which resist expansion, as well as reduce the vertical effect of RPE in hyperdivergent patients. (Michael C[95]., 1987).
7. Edentulous spaces during this period may be treated by an orthodontic appliance to maintain the space for later placement of an implant.

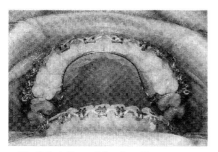

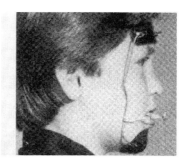

Fig.8.5 A lingual fixed appliance to
maintain the maxillary segments in
the proper position

Fig.8.6 A face mask designed to
help the mandible forward

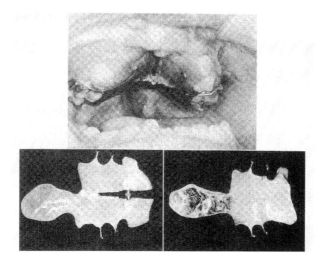

Fig.8.7   A combination appliance for maxillary expansion and obturation of a cleft

8. If edentulous spaces are a hazard to speech production or a source of embarrassment to the child, temporary plates carrying the missing tooth or teeth can be placed.

9. Combined orthodontic and prosthodentic treatment can be done in the late childhood stage to enhance speech and at the same time to obturate the cleft palate (fig.8.7). For example, Lavelle and Van Demark[158] (1976) presented a combination orthodontic – prosthodontic appliance for treatment during the childhood years that incorporated (1) initially a split palatal plate to expand the maxilla with an attached posterior speech bulb to obturate an incompetent velopharyngeal port, which was later modified to become (2) a single anterior palatal plate plus speech bulb.

10. Combined orthodontic and surgical treatment can be done in this late mixed dentition stage. Before eruption of permanent canine in unilateral or bilateral clefts, bone graft is placed to provide continuity of the alveclar arch. Some times it may cause restriction on erupting movement of canine. In this situation that canine may be guided down with a surgically placed orthodontic bracket on the canine tooth surface and an elastic or wire ligature to the orthodontic appliances on the dental arch.

IV. Period of Adult Dentition:

With the final phases of therapy, it becomes apparent that the early stages of therapy involve moving bony palatal segments, while the later stages are usually restricted to individual tooth movement.

Orthodontic management in this period:

1. Extraction of teeth may be recommended to establish a balance between the number and size of dental units and the existing available dental arch length.

    a)   Lower arch crowding can be treated as for non cleft cases. Sometimes the loss of one or more lower incisors can be considered, however, since this has the advantage of reducing the perimeter of the mandibular dental arch anteriorly and thus facilitating the correction of a class III incisor relationship.

    b)   Judicious removal of mandibular first bicuspids may be required to obtain an adequate overbite and overjet relationship of the anterior teeth.

2. Less obviously, it is sometimes possible to change anteroposterior relationship by making adjustments in the vertical dimension. The treatment is based on the observation that in many cleft cases, when the mandible is in the rest position, the skeletal III discrepancy is much reduced and it is only when the patient's teeth are brought into occlusion that an obvious class III occlusion with its associated facial appearance develops. In these cases, it is felt that both upper and lower buccal

segments have failed to erup fully, and there is an increased freeway spare. The condition is associated with a low tongue posture, the tongue lying between the occlusal surfaces of the cheek teeth.

A combination of fixed and removable appliances can be used to extrude the buccal segments so that they contact when the mandible is close to the rest position and thus the excess freeway space is eliminated. The mandible is therefore maintained in a rotated position that masks the skeletal discrepancy.

3. Alignment of the dental arches can be effectively dealt with by using fixed appliance.

4. Abnormal crown root angulations and deficiency of bone in the cleft area can limit the amount of alignment obtainable in some of these patients. Under such circumstances, malalignments must be accepted and the irregularity corrected by crowning.

5. Secondary bone grafting in the cleft site of the anterior maxillary alveolar process may be indicated after the late stages of orthodontic treatment. It enhances facial appearance and helps to stabilize the segments of the maxillary arch and contribute toward maintaining the final orthodontic results.

6. Deficient anteroposterior and vertical growth of the maxilla may be seen in the late adolescent or early adult period. If the maxillomandibular discrepancy is great, midface flatness and mandibular prognathism will develop. A complete cephalometric and clinical evaluation is necessary.

The surgical correction of this abnormality by maxillary advancement and sometimes-mandibular setback requires presurgical orthodontic preparation of the teeth. In this situation the maxillary and mandibular incisors are uprighted and centered over the alveolar ridge. This usually results in an increase in the dental crossbite before surgery. Maxillary and mandibular arch widths are also co-ordinated so that they match correctly upon surgical correction.

Retention is particularly important following many of these cleft treatments where tooth or segment movements place teeth into inherently unstable positions.

ROLE OF PLASTIC SURGEON / ORAL MAXILLO FACIAL SURGEON

Plastic surgeons and maxillofacial surgeons carry out the following surgical treatments:

1. Cleft lip repair
2. Cleft palate repair
3. Surgery to improve velopharyngeal inadequacy

4.   Alveolar bone grafts
5.   Correction of maxillo mandibular disharmonies
6.   Secondary surgical procedures

Treatment of Cleft Lip and Palate:

Aim of treatment of cleft lip and palate is to correct the cleft and associated problems surgically and thus hide the anomaly so that patients can lead normal lives. This correction involves surgically producing a face that does not attract attention, a vocal apparatus that permits intelligible speech and a dentition that allows optimal function and esthetics.

Timing of Surgical Repairs:

The timing of the surgical repairs remains as the most debated issues among the clefts palate team. As surgical correction of the cleft is an elective procedure, if any other medical condition jeopardizes the health of the body, the cleft surgery is postponed until medical risks are minimal, or eliminated.

Normally most surgeons adhere to the rule of 10 for the surgery ie. 10 weeks of age 10 pounds in body weight and at least 10 gm of Hb/dl of blood.

Unfortunately, there are disadvantages besides various advantages in closing a palatal cleft early in life. Advantages are i) better palatal and pharyngeal muscle development once repaired. ii) ease of feeding iii) better development of phonation skills iv) better auditory tube function v) better hygiene when the oral and nasal partition is complete and vi) improved psychologic state for parents and baby.

Disadvantages are; i) surgical correction is more difficult in younger children with small structures and ii) scar formation resulting from the surgery causes maxillary growth restriction.

Although different cleft palate teams time the surgical repair differently a widely accepted principle is compromise.

Lip is closed as early as possible because it has moulding action on the distorted alveolus. Soft palatal cleft is closed between 18-24 months leaving the hard palate open. Hard palatal cleft is then closed in the preschool years around age 4 or 5 as significant maxillary growth has occurred. In between the period of the soft palate and hard palate closure, patient is asked to wear removable palatal obturators.

The mager problem in evaluation of treatment regimens is the fact that the final results of surgical repair of clefts can be judged conclusively by the time the individual's growth is complete[113].

CHEILORRHAPHY

Cheilorrhaphy is the surgical correction of the lip deformity (cheilo – lip, rhaph- junction by a seam or suture).

Objectives:

i) Cheilorrhaphy should restore the functional arrangement of the orbicularis oris musculature to reestablish the normal function of the upper lip.

ii) Cheilorrhaphy should produce a lip that displays normal anatomic structures such as a vermilion tubercle, Cupid's bow and philtrum. Also lip must be symmetric, well contored, soft and supple, and the scars must be inconspicuous.

Surgical techniques:

There are countless techniques as each is unique (fig.8.8). A key point in design is to break up lines of scar, so that fibrosis and contractrue deformity of the lip will be minimized. Chilorrhaphy procedures serve to restore symmetry not only to the lip but also to the nasal tip as well. With the cleft extending through the floor of the nose, the continuity of the nasal apparatus is disrupted. Without the bony foundation for the alar cartilage, a collapse of the lateral aspect of the nose occurs. When the lip is closed, it is necessary to advance this laterally displaced tissue towards the midline. Thus cheilorrhaphy is the first and one of the most important steps in correcting the nasal deformity so common in cleft patients. Various techniques of cleft lip correction are:

1. Le Mesurier technique for incomplete unilateral cleft
2. Tennison operation
3. Millard operation
4. Wynn operation
5. Straight line closure (Veau III operation)
6. Manchester method
7. Skoog method
8. Primary Abbe flap
9. Barsky technique
10. Method of Mulliken
11. Method of Black
12. Method of Noordhoff

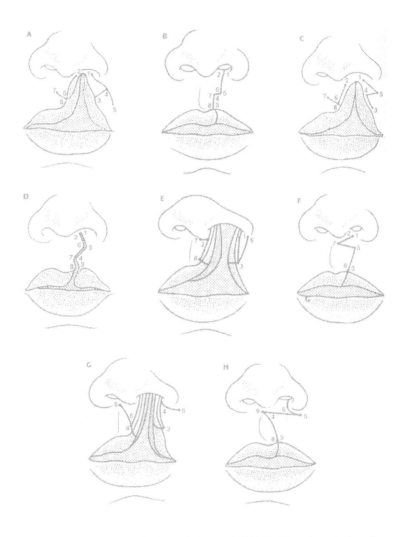

Fig.8.8 Several cheilorrhaphy techniques. A & B, Le Mesurier technique for incomplete unilateral cleft C & D, Tennison operation, E & F, Wynn Operation, G&H

90

Complications of Cheilorrhaphy:

Wound infections
Wound disruption or spreading of scar
Tilting or retrusion of premaxilla
Whistle deformity
Excessively long lip
Collapse of maxillary segments behind premaxilla

Palatorrhaphy

Palatorrhaphy is the surgical correction of the cleft palate deformity. Palatorrhaphy may be performed in one operation or two. In two operations the soft palate closure (Staphylorrhaphy) is usually performed first and the hard palate closure (Uranorrhaphy) is performed second.

Objectives:
The primary purpose of the cleft palate repair is to creat a mechanism capable of speech and deglutition without significantly interfering with subsequent maxillary growth. Thus creation of a competent of the nasal and oral cavity is prerequisites to achieving these goals. The aim is to obtain a long and mobile soft palate capable of producing normal speech.

Surgical Techniques:
Each cleft palate is unique and they vary in width, completeness, amount of hard and soft tissue available and palatal length.

Hard Palate Closure:
Von Langenbeck Operation:

The hard palate is closed with soft tissues only. Usually no effort is made to create an osseous partition between the nasal and oral cavities. The soft tissues extending around the cleft margin vary in their quality. Normally the soft tissues are incised along the cleft margin and dissected from the palatal shelves until approximation over the cleft defect is possible. This procedure usually needs the use of lateral relaxing incisions close to the dentition. The soft tissue are then sutured in a watertight manner over the cleft defect and allowed to heal. The areas of bone exposed by lateral relaxing incisions are allowed to heal by secondary intention (fig.8.9). The superior aspect of the platal flaps will also reepithelialize with respiratory epithelium since this surface is now the lining of the nasal floor. When possible, it is advisable to obtain a two layer closure of the hard platal cleft which necessitates that the nasal mucosa from the floor, lateral wall and septal areas of the nose be mobilized and sutured together before the oral closure. This technique can be modified for concomitant closure of hard and soft palate (fig.8.10).

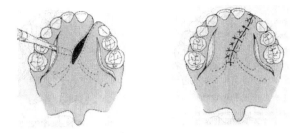

Fig. 8.9 Von langenbeck operation for closure of hard palate

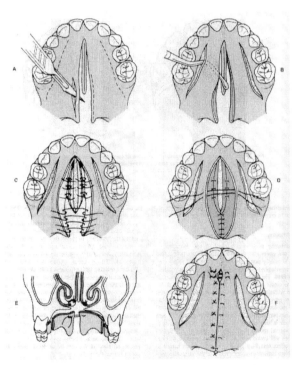

Fig. 8.10 Variation of Von Langenbeck operation for
concomitant hard and soft palate closure

Vomer flap Technique:

When the vomer is long and attached to the palatal shelf opposite the cleft, a mucosal flap can be raised from it and sutured to the palatal tissues on the cleft side. This procedure requires little stripping of palatal mucoperiosteum and produces minimal scar contraction (fig.8.11)

The denuded area of vomer and the opposite sides of the flap where no epthelium is present will reepithelialize. This technique is useful in clefts that are not wide and where the vomer is readily available for use.

Soft Palate Closure:

The closure of the soft palate is technically the most difficult of the operations yet discussed in the cleft–afflicted individual. Access is the largest problem, because the soft palate is toward the back of the oral carity.

Soft palate is always closed in three layers–nasal mucosa muscle and oral mucosa in that order. The margins of the cleft are incised from the posterior end of the hard palate to atleast the dital end of the uvula. The nasal mucosa is then dissected free from the underlying muculature and sutured to the nasal mucosa of the opposite side (fig.8.12).

The muscular layer requires special care. The musculature of the cleft soft palate is not inserted across to the opposite side but instead is inserted posteriorly and laterally along the margins of the hard palate. These muscular insertions must be released from their bony insertions and reapproximated to those of the other sides, only then will the velopharyngeal mechanism have a chance to perform properly.

In cases like short soft palate and articulation with the pharyngeal wall is impossible, i) W-Y push back / wardill procedure ii) U shaped push back / dorrance and Brown procedures are used commonly.

Complications of Palatorrhaphy:

1. Profound bleeding from wound area
2. Airway obstruction and obstructive apnoea
3. Dehiscence
4. Oronasal Fistula

Correction of Velopharyngiel Insufficiency:

Augmentation Pharyngoplasty:
    This technich is an attempt to bring the posterior pharyngeal wall forward, creating tha equivalent of an adenoid pad.

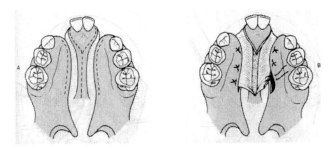

Fig. 8.11 Vomer flap technique for closure of hard palate cleft

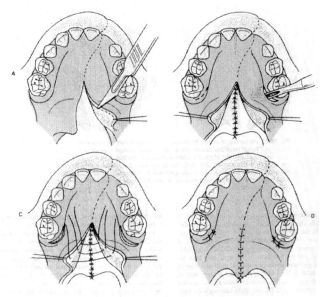

Fig. 8.12 Triple-layered soft palate closure

Advantages:

1. It reproduces the velopharyngeal physiology that would have been in place if the cleft had not occurred. In contrast, most forms of pharyngoplasty attempt to achieve closure by mechanisms that are not as physiologically natural.

2. In addition, if a velar augmentation procedure does not achieve the desired result, the surgeon and team have the option of trying a surgical rearrangement of the pharyngeal musculature.

The techniques that have been used include,

       (1) soft tissue advancement,

       (2) implanting cartilage, and

       (3) injecting or implanting various types of synthetic materials.

1) Soft Tissue Advancement:

Hynes (1950) created an elevation on the posterior pharyngeal wall by dissecting the salpingopharyngeus and its overlying mucosa, lifting these two lateral flaps and suturing them into a pocket he created on the posterior pharyngeal wall by making an incision just below the Eustachian tube orifice. He later modified this procedure to include the palatopharyngeus, salpingopharyngeus, and a portion of the superior constrictor (Hynes, 1953, 1967). He surgically closed the large lateral defects created by the lifting of the lateral flaps; a maneuver that he felt helped to decrease the overall size of the velopharynx.

A recent report by Witt et al., (1997) on "autogenous posterior pharyngeal wall augmentation" invoved the use of a rolled, superiorly based myomucosal flap to create extra thickness on the posterior pharyngeal wall for patients with small velopharyngeal defects.

Cartilage Implants:

Autogenous cartilage (usually from the patient's rib) is used to create an anterior projection or pad on the pharyngeal wall. The implants should be about three times the size of the measured gap in order to produce normal resonance and articulation.

Synthetic Materials:

Mateials that have been used in attempts to move the posterior pharyngeal wall forward include,

- Injectable or implantable forms of silicone or Silastic (Blocksma, 1963, 1964; Brauer, 1973)
- Teflon implants or injections (Ward, Sroudt, and Goldman, 1967)
- Proplast implants (Wolford, Oelschlaeger, and Deal, 1989).
- Most recently, injectable collagen (Remacle et al., 1990).

Sphincter Pharyngoplasty:

Hynes (1953, 1967) stated that his pharyngoplasty could work in any of three ways: by advancing the posterior pharyngeal wall, by reducing the overall diameter (specifically the lateral dimensions) of the pharynx in a static manner, or by producing an active sphincter. Although he did not use the word "sphincter" in his publications, he described the ridge he created as "very prominent and often contractile" (Hynes, 1950), and his work served as the foundation for later innovators who tried to get the velopharynx to work in a sphincteric fashion.

Orticochea (1968, 1970) is the name most frequently associated with sphincter pharyngoplasty. He dissected the posterior faucial pillars from their inferior attachments and the lateral pharyngeal wall and sutured them to an inferiorly based pharyngeal flap.

Modifications were suggested by Jackson and Silverton (1977) whereby the constructed sphincter provides dynamic and static obturation of the velopharyngeal isthmus. This popular technique awaits long-term assessment of its efficacy compared with the pharyngeal flap technique.

ALVEOLAR CLEFT BONE GRAFTING:

Bone grafting of the alveolus has become an essential part of the contemporary surgical management of many orofacial cleft deformities.
Timings of Bone Grafting:

1. Primary bone grafting is undertaken at the age of two years or younger than two years.
2. Early secondary bone graftng is undertaken at the age in between two and five years.
3. Secondary bone grafting is undertaken at the age of five or greater than five years.

Aim of Primary Bone Grafting:

The principal aim in primary alveolar grafting is to prevent significant transverse maxillary collapse and occlusal distortion between the upper and lower arches.

Advantages:

Idealy, this early stabilization decreases the time period of orthodontic treatment in the transitional and adult dentition periods as well as the eventual need for orthognathic surgery. In addition, the early obliteration of the alveolar oronasal fistula eliminates nasal liquid escape and improves oral hygiene in the preschool and early school periods. With this technique, all complete clefts are fitted a maxillary obturator appliance.

Aim of Secondary Bone Grafting:

The principal aim in secondary bone grafting is to unify the maxilla and create an osseous environment that will support tooth eruption into the arch.

Advantages;

1. Stabilization of the maxillary segments, mainly the premaxilla, in bilateral cleft cases.
2. Bone support for the alar cartilage.
3. Continuity of the alveolar ridge from the creation of new alveolar bone in the cleft area.
4. Continuity of the dental arch, with the possibility of moving teeth through the grafting area.
5. Opportunity for spontaneous or induced eruption of the permanent canine as the periodontium develops.
6. The restoration of alveolar bone height is one of the best benefits of the secondary grafted alveolus. This procedure typically provides greater than 80% root coverage of incisors and cuspids adjacent to the cleft (Long et al[82]., 1996). With such bony coverage, the incidence of periodontal defects and fistulae are decreased and long-term tooth retention is markedly improved.

Graft materials:

The choice of donor site for graft material is overwhelmingly the ilium (fig.8.13) from which ample amounts of cancellous bone tissue can be easily obtained (Boyne and Sands[14], 1972). Particulate bone grafts are superior to cortical or corticocancellous grafts because they are more readily incorporated into the alveolus with the capacity for postoperative remodeling.

The favourable experience with calvarial bone in a variety of craniomaxillofacial sites logically led to its application in alveolar clefts (Wolfe and Berkowitz[165], 1983). This donor source has been reported to offer high rates of success, but the method of its harvest has been shown to significantly affect its transplanted oesteogenic capability (Sadove et al[130], 1990).

Other donor sources have included the tibia (in adults) and the mandibular symphysis. With improved methods of graft harvesting, however, the ilium remains the gold standard for secondary alveolar bone grafting (Boustard[13], 1997).

Surgical Procedure:

Grafts are made into particulate consistency and are packed into the defect once the nasal and palatal mucosas have been closed. The labial mucosa is then closed over the bone graft. Intact mucoperiosteal flaps on each side must cover bone graft placed into the alveolar cleft. This means that flaps of nasal mucusa, platal mucosa and labial mucosa must all be developed and sutured in a tension-free, water tight manner to prevent infection of the graft (fig.8.14).

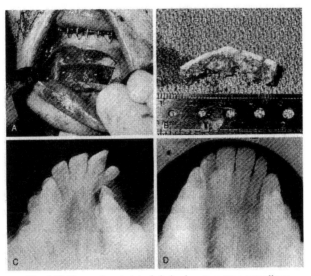

Fig. 8.13 The graft material of choice is autogenous cancellous marrow of the illum

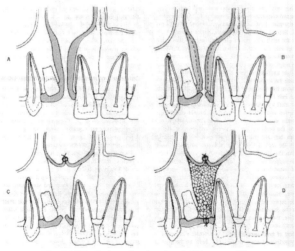

Fig. 8.14 Technique for alveolar cleft bone grafting

In time these grafts are replaced by new bone that is indistinguishable from the surrounding alveolar process. Orthodontic movement of teeth into the graft sites is possible and eruption of teeth into them usually proceeds unimpeded

Correction of maxillo mandibular disharmonies:

Individual with a cleft deformity will usually exhibit maxillary retrusion and a transverse maxillary constriction resulting from the cicatricial contraction of previous surgeries. In many instances it is difficult to correct malocclusion by orthodontic treatment alone. Hence orthognathic surgeries are indicated to correct the skeletal malrelationships.

1. Lefort I Osteotomy

It is the surgical procedure carried out to treat the retruded maxilla by splitting the maxilla from the pterygoid plates and advancing the whole maxilla anteriorly.

2. Distraction Osteogenesis

The process of distraction osteogenesis has been defined as a method of increasing bone length by the controlled daily separation of bone ends on either side of a bone cut. Callus formation occurs 5 to 7 days following the initial bone cuts (latency period). This is followed by bony in–growth as the callus is distracted (activation period). When the required bone length has been achieved, the distraction device remains in place to serve as a rigid skeletal fixation until maturation of the generated new bone is achieved (consolidation period).

This procedure is a viable alternative to conventional osteotomy for patients who have a midface deficiency associated with or without a syndrome or cleft lip and palate.

Secondary surgical procedures:

Secondary surgical procedures are procedures performed after the initial repair of the cleft defects in an effort to improve speech or correct residual defect.

ROLE OF PROSTHODONTIST

Prosthodontic treatment has a long and rich history in the care of patients with cleft lip and palate. Because of increased knowledge of craniofacial growth and development and improved surgical and orthodontic treatment, today's cleft patients receive better care and in less time. This requires less prosthetic intervention. Still, prosthetics retain an important, if somewhat diminished, place in cleft care, and the prosthodontist remains an integral member of the cleft/ craniofacial rehabilitation team.

Premaxilla Positioning Appliance:

The premaxilla-positioning appliance (Reisberg et al., 1988; Figueroa et al., 1996) is a non-surgical technique that retracts and rotates the malposed segment to a more favourable position for lip repair.

A hard resin palatal plate is made from a maxillary impression of the infant. An orthodontic button is attached to the polished surface on each side in the area overlying the gumpads. A 1.0 cm^2- by $-$ 2.0-mm thick pad of soft denture reline material is added to a segment of an elastic orthodontic chain. The ends of the chain are attached to the orthodontic buttons on the plate.

The tissue surface of the palatal plate is lined with resilient denture reline material for intimate soft tissue contact and fit. Denture adhesive is used to help retain the plate in the mouth.

The elastic chain is draped over the premaxillary segment with the soft pad contacting the prolabium. The palatal plate provides anchorage for the elastic chain as it delivers a low–grade, steady traction force of 5.0g on the premaxillary segment.

As the premaxillary segment moves down and back to a more favourable position, the elastic chain can be adjusted at the orthodontic buttons to maintain the desired force on the segment. The anterior portion of the plate needs to be relieved periodically to allow continuous retraction of the premaxilla.

Treatment is continued until the plastic surgeon feels that the premaxilla has been moved to a favourable position for lip repair; usually 2 to 3 months. If the palatal segments are collapsed, an expansion screw can be incorporated into the palatal plate to permit ongoing retraction.

Nasal Conformer:

The nasal cartilages are soft and amenable to moulding for several months after birth responding well to nonsurgical correction using a nasal splint (Matsuo and Hirose[87] 1991).

Grayson et al[58]. (1999) has described the use of a nasal orthopedic moulding appliance to minimize or avoid this problem. A resin palatal plate is made for the infant at 2 to 3 weeks of age. A small projection of resin extends from the plate at the cleft lip site up toward the alar cartilage. This projection is covered with a resilient denture- lining material and makes contact with the cartilage to slightly elevate it and mold it to proper contour. This conformer is retained with denture adhesive and is worn continuously except for daily cleaning until the cleft lip repair. During the period of wear the patient is seen at 1 to 2 week intervals for adjustments.

Articulation Development Prosthesis:

Articulation development prosthesis (Dorf et al., 1985) is used to prosthetically create a normal palate for speech development until the surgical repair can be performed (fig.8.15)

This resin plate covers the gum pads and palate area but does not extend into the cleft. This design permits appositional growth at the cleft margins. This design permits appositional growth at the cleft margins. The prosthesis has a small extension into the pharyngeal area; care must be taken so this is not overextended, or it can cause pharyngeal soft tissue irritation and lack of stability. This prosthesis is retained with denture adhesive and is worn continuously except for cleaning several times a day. The prosthesis will not impede the eruption of teeth, and if any teeth are already present, it can be designed to circumvent them.

Palatal Obturator:

A palatal obturator covers the opening and contributes to normal speech production. It eliminates hypernasality and assists speech therapy for correction of compensatory articulations (fig.8.16).

The prosthesis consists of a resin palatal plate with retention clasps of stainless steel orthodontic wire. The teeth that are clasped may need to be modified so that their shape is more favourable for retaining the clasps. In addition, if any teeth are congenitally missing, they can be attached to the plate to improve articulation and appearance. This prosthesis is often used as an interim measure until the residual communication can be surgically closed. If the oronasal opening cannot be surgically repaired, the palatal obturator may serve as a definitive treatment.

Palatopharyngeal Obturator:

A Palatopharyngeal obturator provides velopharyngeal closure and contributes to normal function. The palatal portion of this resin plate covers the hard palate and is attached to several teeth with wire clasps. This serves to retain and stabilize the prosthesis. The velar portion extends into the pharyngeal area at the level of the palatal plane and seals the nasal cavity from the oropharynx during function. This prosthesis is most often used as an interim device until corrective surgery can be performed. It may serve as the definitive therapy when no further surgery is planned (fig.8.17).

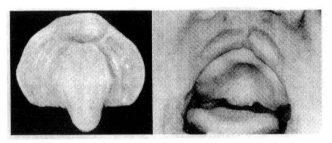

Fig. 8.15: The "articulation development" prosthesis

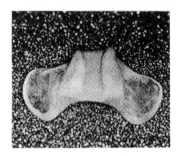

Fig. 8.16 Palatal obturator

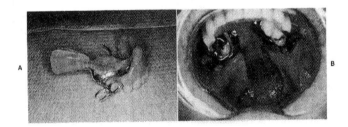

Fig. 8.17 A combination of Palatopharyngeal obturator with
artificial teeth

Palatal Lift:

Velopharyngeal incompetency occurs when the surgically repaired soft palate is of adequate length but of inadequate mobility to elevate to achieve velopharyngeal closure. Palatal lift prosthesis covers the hard palate and extends posteriorly to engage the soft palate and physically elevate and extend it to the proper position to achieve closure. This prosthesis is most effective when the soft palate has little muscle tone and offers little resistance to elevation (fig.8.18).

Tooth Replacement:

Edentulous spaces in which teeth are congenitally missing can be closed orthodontically or surgically during an orthognathic procedure. When the edentulous cleft site is not closed orthodontically or surgically, some type of prosthetic treatment is required.

A removable partial denture is most often used as a temporary form of tooth replacement (fig.8.19). Although it can provide good esthetics, portions of the prosthesis must rest on soft tissues of the palate and can cause irritation. There may be movement of the prosthesis during function. The fact that it is removable accentuates its artificial character, which is a common objection from patients. It is used only as a definitive means of tooth replacement in which there are multiple teeth missing and the edentulous space is too long to be spanned by a fixed restoration.

A conventional fixed partial denture can be used. This requires filing down at least one tooth on each side of the edentulous space and placing a full crown restoration on them. The porcelain artificial tooth is connected to these crowns, which are made of porcelain fused to a metal alloy. The entire fixed tooth replacement of artificial tooth and crowns is cemented over the prepared abutment teeth. Like the resin – bonded prosthesis, function and esthetics are excellent. Long – term success is more predictable.

If adequate volume of bone exists in the edentulous space, tooth replacement can be achieved using dental implants (fig.8.20). A titanium alloy analogue of a tooth root is surgically placed in the bone at the site of the missing tooth. This can be placed in natural bone or at a bone-grafted site. The implant is covered by the soft tissue and heals for 6 months. During this healing period, osseointegration occurs. That is, the bone connects to the implant surface to hold it in place. Then the implant is connected through the oral soft tissue, and a porcelain crown is attached to it. This restores the dental arch to the most natural state, provides excellent function and appearance, and does not require the involvement of adjacent natural teeth.

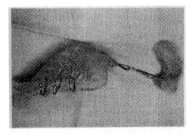 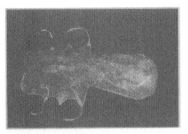

Fig. 8.18 Two different types of palatal lift

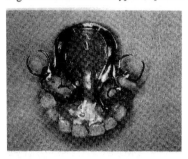

Fig. 8.19 A combination of removable denture + palatal obturator

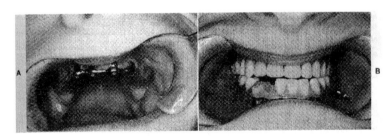

Fig.8.19Stages in treatment of a patient receiving osseointegrated
implants to replace missing teeth

A. The posts have been implanted into the maxillary bone
B. The posts serve as anchors for the replacement teeth in the maxilla

Role of Otolaryngologist:

The otolaryngologists and audiologists who take responsibility for providing optimal ear care for children and adults with clefts are advocating early and continuous otologic surveillance of these patients.

They recommend for early myringotomies and placement of ventilating tubes to the otologic problems associated with cleft.

Early examination of the ears by a qualified otolaryngologist, with prompt evacuation of middle ear fluid and insertion of ventilating tubes or grommets in the tympanic incision, has become routine. This approach, plus the vigilance of the otolaryngologist and the concerned parent aiming to treat middle ear infection early in the process, rather than late, has reduced the incidence of permanent hearing loss, cholesteatoma, tympanic membrane scarring, perforation, and atrophy. Since hearing is so critical for speech production, improved hearing is extremely valuable (Spriestersbach and associates[140], 1962; McWilliams, Morris, and Shelton[94], 1984).

In 1986, Moore, Moore, and Yonkers[100] concluded from their review of literature, "If the lip and palate cannot be repaired by the age of six months, tubes should be placed while waiting for the infant to reach acceptable criteria to allow cleft repair."

Factors Affecting Improvement of Otological Problems

1) Effect of Age Advancement:

There is some evidence that middle ear problem in the infant with a cleft increase in the first few months of life, as they tend to do in infants without clefts. Too-chung (1983) documented normal middle ear function by tympanometry in 84 babies with clefts at birth but middle ear "complications" by the age of 17 weeks. Age continues to be an important variable as the child matures; with a decrease in otologic problems both in cleft and non-cleft children as age increases.

There appears to be an underlying natural tendency for the occurrence of otitis media to decrease as either noncleft or cleft palate children mature. Perhaps this is related to the plane of the eustachian tube becoming more vertical than horizontal as the child grows, improving the muscle vectors for function of the tensor veli palatini, or to an increase in cartilage support of the tube (Blustone et al[12] 1975).

2. Effects of Palatoplasty:

To date, no single technique of palatoplasty has proven universally advantageous to produce better results in terms of eliminating or reducing further ear disease. One area of specific concern has been whether surgery includes fracturing of hamulus to obtain more medial "relocation" of tensor veli palatini and thus facilitate closure of the palate.

Fracturing the hamulus was a frequent part of palatoplasty in the 1960s. When otologists became more routinely involved in the case of babies with cleft palates, voiced their concern about the possible effects of this procedure on the ability of the tensor to open the eustachian tube (Stool[142] 1989). Today most techniques for palatoplasty do not include hamulotomy.

In 1971, Edgerton and Dellon reported that retrodisplacement of the levator (into a more normal position) as a part of palatal repair provided substantial improvement in hearing.

A study conducted by Smith, DiRuggiero, and Jones in 1994, provided data that the improvement in eustachian tube function seen in children with clefts after palate repair may take several years to show up, which immediately raises the question of whether the improvement they found was simply a function of increased age of the child.

In one recent study in which the palatal clefts were closed within the first month of life in 18 children, 13 (72%) still required placement of ventilating tubes sometimes during their first 3 years of life because of persistent or recurrent perfusion (Nunn et al[106]., 1995). The surgical technique in this study was a push back palatoplasty. The author concluded that early palate closure did not significantly alter the need for myringotomy and tubes in children with clefts.

The impression gained in reviewing the studies of the effects of palatal closure on subsequent ear disease is that surgical closure alone is not enough to optimize otologic health and that ventilation tubes are required.

Complications of the ventilating tubes:

(i) Regurgitation of fluids through tubes into the outer ear canal if the palate has not been closed.

ii) Permanent tympanic membrane perforation and scarring. (Braganza et. Al[15]., 1991, Rynnel – Dagoo et al[129]. 1992).

Role of Speech Therapist

The speech pathologist functions essentially as a monitor of speech output. All speech sounds are analyzed to determine deviations from normal, and the cause of any deviation is evaluated. To the extent that anatomic variations are corrected, the speech pathologist offers therapeutic options to enhance maturation of speech or to achieve satisfactory compensation in motor production for optimal speech.

The use of instruments is essential in the evaluation and documentation of velopharyngeal function. The instruments described below have proven clinical and research value for assessing velopharyngeal valving. Instrumentation for assessing velopharyngeal mechanism includes,

1. Radiography – (Towne's view)
2. Cinefluoroscopy and videofluoroscopy
3. Nasal endoscopy and oral endoscopy
4. Pressure–flow technique
5. Nasometer
6. Accelerometers
7. Spectrography
8. Photodetection
9. Electromyography
10. Acoustic rhinometry
11. Electropalatography

The majority of children referred for therapy typically require intervention to enhance their articulation or phonological development or general expressive language functioning. Although the course of speech therapy will be very straightforward for some children, it will be far more complex for others who demonstrate articulation and resonance problems associated with velopharyngeal incompetence.

1. Early Intervention Programming:

Initially the primary role of a speech language pathologist working on a cleft palate team will be one of parent education. Parents are often unsure of what the impact of the cleft will be and thus are uncertain of what they should expect of the child.

Parents of babies with cleft palate should be informed of the impact that a cleft has on a child's oropharyngeal mechanism and how this may be expected to affect the child's early communicative efforts as well as speech production performance after palatoplasty. In addition to counseling parents about the expected impact of the cleft on speech the clinician will also want to encourage aggressive language stimulations.

It is not uncommon for these children to experience delays in speech and development and expressive language. Before palatal surgery parents should be encouraged to engage the child in vocal play and babbling games (just as they would with any infant). They should be informed that nasal consonants and glides will be more easily and perhaps more readily produced than pressure consonants. However approximation of pressure consonants should always be accepted despite any distortion that may be present.

Compensatory articulations, particularly aberrant glottal behaviours, should be described and the parents counseled to avoid reinforcing them. Instead of repeating that "cute' growl to the baby, parents should be encouraged to simply ignore these undesired behaviors when they are produced but reinforce the baby's efforts to vocalize by producing a babble or word that contains desired consonants. Parents should also be encouraged to monitor the different consonants that the child produces while babbling.

According to Bzoch (1997) an optimal programme would include:
<ul>
<li>i)   parent counseling regarding language development,</li>
<li>ii)   home speech and language stimulations programme,</li>
<li>iii)   direct speech therapy when indicated,</li>
<li>iv)   team management approach involving the plastic surgeon and a dental specialist in each community.</li>
</ul>

2. Direct Articulation–Phonological Therapy:

The type of therapy and the frequency of therapy should be based on each child's individual needs. A child who is demonstrating a general delay in language development may well benefit from enrollment in a classroom – based intervention programme. A child with intelligible speech who demonstrates developmental substitution errors may indeed benefit from direct speech therapy provided only one a week. However a child with CP who demonstrates poor consonant development or compensatory articulation errors will likely require more intensive intervention to establish normal oral articulation in a reasonable period of time.

In general, the speech therapists recommend use of long–standing therapy techniques for teaching children to produce sounds in syllabus and words and then establishing automatic use of those sounds in conversation. Therapy should include use of auditory and visual models for imitation, practice and reinforcement of responses in age – appropriate speech material and should be organized to encourage generalization from that which is taught in therapy to speech units not used in therapy and to situations outside the clinic.

Initiating articulation therapy for some young children with CP who demonstrates evidence of velopharyngeal inadequacy can be difficult when they make no effort to use their oral articulators to create labial and lingual constrictions to stop or modulate air flow.

Blowing tasks are useful with young children in teaching the concept of oral airflow. However they are not very useful in teaching consonant productions.

Although blowing tasks can be used to heighten awareness of oral airflow, they should never be considered a therapy goal.

Oral motor "exercises" are introduced on the assumption that lack of oral articulation reflects an underlying problem with muscle strength. Unfortunately, the majority of children with CP who are subjected to these treatment strategies do not benefit from them because there is no underlying neuromotor problem to begin with.

3. Therapy for Poor Consonant Development

Children with CP who demonstrate poor consonant development in the absence of significant cognitive and receptive language delays, hearing loss, or neurological problems are challenging management cases for the speech language pathologist who serves in a cleft palate team.

The appropriate management in cases like this is therapy to eliminate the nasal and glottal substitutions and establish oral articulations. Surgical management should not be considered until the child is attempting production of pressure consonants and there is evidence of velopharyngeal inadequacy.

The rapid eleimination of nasal substitutions and co articulated glottal stops reported by Broen, Doyle, and Bacon (1993) after placement of a speech bulb was very impressive. Unfortunately, not all centers offer prosthetic management as an adjunct to treatment. This speech bulb can be used to control velopharyngeal inadequacy in young children.

4. Dental Malocclusion and Oral Distortions:

Dental occlusal problems frequently compromise articulatory precision in children with CP and result in oral distortion. Children with a severe class II malocclusion may be unable to approximate lips for adequate production of bilabial consonants. So, production of these consonants must be accomplished by labiodental articulation. Children with severe class III malaclusion may be obligated to produce some lingua–alveolar consonants using interdental placement.

It denotes the combined orthodontic and speech therapy treatment is needed to remove the dental cause of the speech problem.

Phoneme–Specific Nasal Emission

Most clinicians address the problem of phoneme specific nasal emission by using a facilitating sound to elicit oral production of the target sound. For example, /t/ is a sound that shares the same place of production as /s/. When a child who produces a /t/ (that is free of nasal emission) is instructed to produce a series of /t/ s and prolong the last one (eg. "T...T...t...Sssssss) the result will be an oral /s/. A word of caution here the target sound in this example is a "long" /t/ not a /s/. It is important to instructing the child to produce a long /t/ not an (s) because the latter sound is associated with nasal emission in the child's mind. Referring to the target sound as "s" can, and initially probably will elicit nasal emission.

Riski [124](1984) recommended placing a straw in front of the patient's mouth to increase the perceptual awareness of oral turbulence. Other types of auditory and visual feedback that may be helpful in eliminating phoneme specific nasal emission include the use of simple devices such as a See Scape and a listening tube-stethoscope.

Witzel, Tobe, and Salyer[164] (1988) recommended the use of nasopharyngoscopy as a biofeed back tool. Ruscello, Schuster and Sandwisch 1991 described a programme to eliminate context specific nasal emission with a combination of biofeed back and articulation therapy.

Compensatory Articulation:

Glottal and pharyngeal articulations are often difficult to eliminate in young children. This is true whether they occur in an individual with past or present velopharygeal inadequacy. Because these maladaptive patterns are a typical and they can have more serious consequences for speech intelligibility than other developmental substitutions that the child may be producing. Thus, it is often advisable to address these errors in therapy before addressing other substitution errors.

Glottal Stops:

These laryngeal productions are generally addressed by having a patient whisper the target sound and produce an aspirate /h/ after it to break up the glottal pattern. It is typically recommended that voiceless stops be addressed before voiced stops.

When attempting to eliminate glottal stop substitutions for labial and lingual stops, the patient is generally instructed to sustain /h/ as lips open and close for production of /p/ or /t/. The patient is instructed to over aspirate the stop consonant before gradually adding voicing for the vowel. When attempting to eliminate glottal stop substitutions for velar stops, instruct the patient to produce the velar nasal (n) while the parents occlude the child nares. The result will be a velar stop. The patient can be encouraged to over aspirate the stop consonant using /h/.

It is often easier to eliminate compensating articulation and establish an oral stop by first training a voiceless homorganic oral fricative (Trost, 1981).

Pharyngeal Fricatives or Stops

These atypical patterns of articulation can be eliminated by use of anterior facilitating sound to elict the target sound. For example, if a child substitutes a voiceless paryrgeal fricative for an /s/, /s/ can be elicited by having the child produce a series of /t/s followed by a prolonged /s/ (et., t...t...sssssssssss). When a pharyngeal fricative is coorticulation either an unaspirated continuant or a stop can be used to stimuate the target sound (Trost – Cardoamone, 1995). Other articulating postures that have been recommended to facilitate production of /s/ include /o/ and /ʃ/. The patient is instructed to initiate oral air flow for /o/ and then gradually retract the tongue to a postdental position while maintaining oral airflow.

Trost – Cardamone noted that the high, front vowel /i/ can also facilitate anterior placement. She recommended the use of ortho elastics and cereal bits placed on the tongue to facilitate phonetic placements.

Midddorsum Palatal Stops

The goal of therapy when eliminating middorsum platal stops is to establish the lingua-alveolar place of production and or the velar place of production. As with other atypical articulations, the place feature should be established first before the stop manner is addressed. Trost–Cardomone (1995) observed that homorganic /n,l/ and /s,z/ can be helpful in teaching the appropriate placement for linguaalveolar stops. A word of caution: when a palatal fistula is present, these substitution errors may be more easily eliminated after surgical closure or obstruction of the fistula.

Therapy for Persons with Velopharyngeal Inadequacy:

Surgical management of obstruction can be done, but any speech therapy provided to these patients is not expected to establish normal speech. Rather the goal is to help the patient do as well as possible. Speech pathologist should avoid asking these patients to produce sounds with good oral air pressure because such efforts may encourage the gross substitutions that therapy is intended to correct.

Strategies to reduce perceived nasalization like (a) Increasing mouth opening to promote an increase in oral resonance (Boone and Mc Farlane[21], 1994),
(b) Use of light articulatory contacts to decrease listener perception of audible nasal emission (Van Demark and Hardin[158], 1990), (c) Reducing the speech rate (most controversial technique) may also be used.

Strategies to improve velopharyngeal function:
i. Muscle training
    Eg: Continuos Positive Air Pressure Therapy (CPAP) (Kaehn[71] 1991) and Whistling Blowing Technique (Shprintzen, Mcall and Skolnick (1975).

ii. Information feedback
    Eg: Endoscopy,
             Aeromechanical measures,
             Auditory recordings,
             Electromyography.
iii. Obturators
    Eg: speech bulb prosthesis.

Role of Psychiatrist / Psychologist

The psychiatrist and psychologist evaluate the patient for strengths and weakness in cognitive, interpersonal, emotions, behavioral, and social development. Emphasis is placed on the patient's ability to cope with the emotional and physical stress created by the cleft defect. Consolation with the parents and schools regarding educational or behavioral management is carried out when indicated.

Broder and Strauss[19] (1989) also urged routine psychosocial screening by teams and preventive psychosocial intervention to help these children develop their potential and to improve behavioral adjustment. Tobiasen[148] (1990) strongly urged that at least one psychological assessment be completed for every child with a cleft before entrance into school and repeated every 2 to 3 years thereafter. She also recommended that older children and their parents should routinely be offered consultations with a psychologist before and after each major surgery. In 1991, Strauss and Broder stressed the need of mental health workers to develop support groups for families, provide nursing and feeding instruction, dispense literature to enlighten family members and school personnel about cleft conditions, assess patients and family systems, and provide counseling to patients and their families.

Kapp – Simon and Simon (1991) devised a hands-on social skills training program for teenagers with craniofacial anomalies, designed to teach them how to handle difficult social situations, deal with pesky peers, and maintain a healthy and balanced attitudes as they mature through these difficult years.

Peterson and falzon (1999) mentioned that the push for preventive measures and intervention with regard to psychosocial problems in individuals with clefts came into toe – to – toe opposition with the 1990s' push for minimizing costs of care by reducing that care to the lowest possible level. When psychologists and other mental health care professionals first had an opportunity to examine and counsel these patients and their families in the 1950s' 1960s', and 1970s' many craniofacial teams were funded by federal grants that supported the interdisciplinary approach to treatment. Sadly that was no longer the case. As we left the 1900s' we knew more than we had ever known about these needs and have fewer resources to meet them than our predecessors had in previous decades.

Role of Nurse

Ideally, the first person to consult with the parents of a newborn with a cleft should be a feeding specialist, usually the nurse on the team.

One of the most important functions of the team nurse as a consultant is to provide outreach education and coordination with community hospitals, especially newborn nurseries or neonatal intensive care units, as well as with paediatricians and community health clinics. This is critical at the time of birth or when the diagnosis is made in order to provide health care providers with accurate information and speciality expertise.

Another aspect of the nurse's consultant role can be described as "patient and family advocate". In this role, the nurse serves as a liaision to nursing staff, craniofacial team members, primary health care providers, and community agencies. For example, to the nursing staff in the paediatric unit, a mother may seem overly anxious and concerned about feeding her infant after surgery and the possibility of weight loss. Nurses and staff support personnel may be more emphathetic if they understand the initial problems and frustrations that the mother experiences when feeding her newborn and how weight gain is an important milestone.

Additional educational responsibilities of the craniofacial nurse include ongoing staff education of hospital – based nursing personnel who care for these families, as well as of nursing students or other health care providers. This education may extend into public areas such as the school system, community organizations or government agencies.

A comparatively new aspect of the nurse's role is in the area of research that includes the proper feeding method and weight gain, postoperative feeding techniques and pain management as well as a variety of psychosocial issue (TimorthyA Turvay[147],1996) .

Treatment for Feeding Problem:

Mother should have been stressed to take over as many feedings as possible. A different nurse should carry those that she cannot do out if possible each time. In this way the mother soon masters the little details given by the feeding specialists, becomes the real expert in feeding her child, and realizes that she is the most important person in keeping the child alive.

The importance of early "bonding" particularly when the child has a facial deformity cannot be overstressed. Often, however, the oldest and most experienced nurse in the nursery literally "takes over" the feeding "problem" and willingly relieves the anxious mother of this additional burden. This seperates the mother and child at a critical time in a basic need and function, and should be avoided if at all possible.

Commonly used devices and Techniques:

i)   A standard bottle with enlarged (1/4 inch) cross cut regular nipple and Mead Johnson cleft palate Nurser are the most commonly used devices for the feeding problem of cleft lip and palate patients.

ii)   The so-called "Cleft palate nipple" with a rubber flange to obturate the cleft rarely if ever, proves satisfactory. The child should take a full feeding in about 30 minutes; if it takes longer, the child probably is working too hard to eat.

iii)   The child should be held at a 45-degree angle or semi-upright position instead of supine position, so that less milk escapes into the nasal passages. The ability to swallow is not usually impaired. The child with a cleft palate can be expected to swallow more than the usual amount of air, and requires more than the usual amount of "burping".

iv)   The direct breast feeding has not usually been successful; however, a breast pump may permit a motivated mother to provide breast milk for her infant.

v)   The use of soft-sided "squeezable bottles" and soft nipples perhaps with enlarged holes, and into the noncleft side of the palate or in bilateral clefts, against the larger palatine shelfwill help the child in feeding.

vi)   The use of silastic bifid cleft palate nipple designed by Kanneth Adisman (1957) is also recommended.

vii)   The modified Hotz–Type plate is an acrylic plate covering the palatal surface of cleft palate with an acrylic ridge along the posterior edge of the hard palate. This ridge made tight contact with the dorsal surface of the tongue and occluded the oropharyngeal airway during suckling.
Mikihiko Kago[96] (1997) concluded that three factors must be addressed for CL /CP patients to facilitate successful breast feeding: (1) close the cleft in the lip (2) close the cleft in the hard palate and (3) make tight contact between the tongue and posterior palate.
The palatal ridge on the Hotz-type plate cut off the connection with the upper airway when the tongue was pressed toward the ridge.

viii)   The combined use of a palatal obturator, Haberman bottle, and breast milk pumping, and lactation education is very successful in increasing intake and reducing time to feed. It also enhances good growth in patients with CP. (Leslie Turner et al[81]., 2001)

Role of primary care physician:

Primary care physicians have a vital role for families of children with cleft lip, cleft palate, or both. Physicians should provide proper information at a time when parents have questions; they should address the physical and psychological issues that arise.

The new born period is one of the most important and difficult times for a family and the primary physician may be of great assistance to these families. Parents of infants with clefts are usually shocked and confused (Woar 1991). Parents have stated that one of the most stressful situations is to be isolated without interaction by staff during the initial days following birth. Also, misinterpretation of information can be very devasting and long lasting (Mc Donald, 1979).

Parents are often poorly informed and have incorrect information and superstitions regarding a child with a cleft (Woar, 1991). Too often feeding issues take priority over the parents, need for support and proper information (Curtin, 1990). Well-informed parents have been shown to have less stress with such issues. Parent's fears need to be addressed and parents ideally should be connected as soon as possible, perhaps within 24 hours of birth, to a cleft care multidisciplinary team (Yetter 1992; Hatel et al, 1996), although surgery may occur for several weeks after birth. The primary physician can be an important for parents' adjustment during the time interval before the initial cleft palate center visit.

Primary care physician's role can be invaluable when dealing with such as issues of feeding, developmental delays, behavior problems, and recurrent infections (Kaufman 1991). Besides advising team members about family medial history and medical allergies, they can be the best patient advocates (Kaufman, 1991). Physicians must not see treatment of clefts as a simple closure of a wound but as a birth defect with lifelong physical, social, and psychological effects.

Physician can be a helpful link between the families and the multidisciplinary team. He needs to be knowledgeable about the cleft team concept and its importance. This should be included in the medical update.

Physicians have the responsibility of providing education, answers and comfort to the parents. Physicians from craniofacial cleft centers must assist primary physician with appropriate referrals for newborns with a cleft. They have the responsibility of helping parents to enjoy and do the best for their children. (Jennifer L.Gron[67], 2002)

Role of Geneticist:

Genetic Counseling:

Information about heredity, all too often incorrect, has been provided for families with children showing unusual congenital defects since the development of communication. The advice of friends, enemies, and neighbors in many instances has been effective in altering reproductive behaviour of the family in question. Although such illfounded advice has precedent in time, in our modern society we like to believe that enlightened attitudes and accurate information will avoid such mystical approches to science. Since advice about heredity will inevitably be sought and given, it would seem that the professional geneticist is in a better position to give it than even one's best friend. This brings us to the consideration of the requirements for a counselor in hereditary problems.

First of all, this person must have a working knowledge of human genetics. Genetic of inheritance, gene interaction in families and human populations, and chromosomal abnormalities with all of their consequences is a few of the important subjects to be comprehended by the genetic counselor. With this armamentarium, facts and figures can be sorted out and presented intelligently to the people being counseled.

The second and perhaps equally important requirement for a genetic counselor is a deep respect for the attitudes, sensitivities, and reaction of the people being counseled. It is not enough to make a diagnosis and then lay out the bare facts of the problem. Admittedly, such facts are unusally presented in some detail and are only rarely withheld but the framework in which they are presented is very important. Only when the counselor knows that the facts are understood and are not being distorted by the patients – either consciously or unconsciously-can he or she assume that a service is being done. Feelings of guilt, fear, hostility, and resentment are frequently encountered at the counseling table. A mother of newborn child with a cleft lip and palate may suddenly find herself rejected by her husband when he retrospectively discovers that her great-uncle was similarly afflicted. This husband may come to the counselor convinced that a"bad gene" presented on his wife's side of the family has been concealed from him. Only after a careful discussion of the nongenetic causes of cleft lip and palate, the frequent failure of individuals who carry genetic traits to show them, and the prospective or empiric risks of two normal parents having children afflicted with any congenital abnormality can the genetic counselor finally communicate the nature of the problem to the clients.

Finally, the genetic counselor must have a sincere desire to teach the truth to the full extent that it is known. By careful attention to responses, the feedback necessary for evaluation of success in communication can be obtained, a technique used by all good teachers.

Prenatal Parental Counseling:

The advancing sophistication and availability of prenatal diagnostic techniques, such as transvaginal ultrasound, chorionic villus sampling, amniocentesis, and alpha feto–protein testing, have increased the medical capacity to detect genetic and congenital conditions during pregnancy.

The prenatal diagnosis of a congenital defect marks the beginning of a period of high stress and uncertainity for many parents. When people receive bad news, they experience a loss of control and are in crisis. This may be a time when parents are vulnerable and are easily swayed by the opinion of professionals or other parents. Prospective parents should be carefully informed of all of their possible options and afforded time to make their decision. In the prenatal period, prospective parents should receive nonjudgemental and unbiased information, support, and advice from health professionals who are specifically trained to counsel and support decisions. Family physicians and other professionals with a continuous relationship with the family would be ideal counselors at this time of considerable parental stress. In a paper by Jones (1999), the presentation of information to families was described in a positive way, with good achievable outcomes.

The establishment of optimism and hope around a cronifacial diagnosis may be a critical step in starting the process of treatment and care, even during the prenatal period [Ronald P. Strauss[126] (2002)].

Role of Social Workers

The social worker acts as the patient's advocate in many cases and aids in psychosocial assessment. This team member assists the family by making referrals to persons or agencies on the local, county to persons or agencies on the local, county, and state levels for guidance regarding financial resources for the patient's medical care. During hospitalization, the social workers provide supportive counseling and facilitate communication between the family and medical or hospital personnel. The focus is on helping the family to cope with stress during and after surgery and to deal with emotional factors involved in forming realistic expectations of surgical outcomes and in adapting to problems of body image.

Examples of some associations formed to provide help to the cleft lip and palate patients.
    1. CLAPAI
    2. The Smile Train
    3. ACPA

CLAPAI

1.   The Cleft Lip and Palate Association of Ireland (CLAPAI) was inaugurated in 1981 to serve the interests of cleft palate individuals and families. It Provides

- Information and support for patients parents
- Funding of vital equipment for hospitals
- Seminars involving parents and the medical profession
- Grants for medical staff and students to enhance knowledge
- Booklets and pamphlets.

CLAPAI seeks to provide support through talking to new parents and providing advice on feeding, and ongoing medical care throughout the treatment. Most of the people active on the CLAPAI committee are parents themselves, and thus are in a position to give `a valuable perspective, practical advice and support. It has also been active in fund-raising in order to aid, hospitals and clinics in the purchase of new equipment, and has assisted in sending medical professionals to conferences abroad.

In addition, the association has played a prominent role in the formulation and development of government and medical policy and the resultant level of medical services, which were spartan initially, are now vastly improved, always with scope for improvement. Efforts in recent years have included revitalising the organization as a national entity, ensuring that the association acts as a unified group, and devising and implemeting administrative structures for the future in keeping with a national charitable organization.

1. The Smile Train

The Smile Train was started to bring smiles to the face of children with CL/CP, and is a united states–based non-governmental organization, operates in 25 countries. And, it provides assistance to each and every child born with a cleft lip and palate who cannot afford surgical repair.

The Smile Train is unique in its comprehensive approach to cleft lip and palate care by offering free treatment for children, free training for doctors and funding of research efforts to find causes and cures for cleft.

In US the smile train has joined forces with the American Cleft Palate – Craniofacial Association/Cleft Palate Foundation (ACPA) to help provide assistance to children in the US that are born with cleft lip and palate. The Smile Train and ACPA are collaborating on a number of areas, including the complete support of CLEFTLINE, (1-800-24 cleft) a toll-free number. More than 5,000 people call the toll free number for help every year. Through their partnerships with numerous organizations that are dedicated to helping children born with clefts, the Smile Train helps deliver smiles in 40 countries around the world.

Recently, The Smile Train announced five new partnerships with various Indian organizations that will provide more than 12,000 children with cleft lip and palate surgeries over the next three years.

Chapter-9

CONCLUSION

Surveillance studies have shown that cleft lip and palate (CL/CP) is one of the commonest craniofacial anomalies (CFA), occurring in approximately 1 in 500 live births. Taking into consideration the world population and annual birth rates. it is estimated that there are well over a quarter million babies born each year with CL/P. The cost of managing this huge number of clefts is enormous and exceeds the available resources of most developing countries. Thus, CL/CP constitutes a major health problem, which requires globally based strategies to deal with the issues of epidemiology, primary prevention and treatment strategies, which are evidence-based, and cost-effective[171].

Basic research to unravel the etiological factors responsible for clefting disorders is occurring on a worldwide scale, especially in the areas of molecular genetics and gene-environment interactions. There are also in place international organizations such as the WHO Task Force on CFA, the International Consortium on Oral Cleft Genetics (ICOCG), Interplast and other international volunteer cleft missions to help in the treatment of patients with cleft disorders in developing countries, in data collection, in pooling of genetic material and sharing of information. However, there is an urgent need for more randomised clinical trials (RCTs) to evaluate the outcomes of treatment so that clinical guidelines and treatment protocols are based on strong evidence.

BIBLIOGRAPHY

1. Alexandra Sarzyla Medeiros et al. Prevalence of intranasal ectopic teeth in children with complete unilateral and bilateral cleft lip and palate. Cleft Palate Craniofac J.2000: 37; 271 – 274.

2. A Cameron and R Widmer. Handbook of Pediatric dentisitry, 1997, 289-305.

3. ACPA – Clinical guideline on patients with cleft lip/palate and other craniofacial anomalies. American Acadamy of Pediatric Dentistry J. 2000:65-66.

4. AHR ROWE et al, A comprehensive guide to clinical Densitry, 1st edi. 1995; 1317-1347.

5. Andrew C. Lindral et al. Studies of the candidate genes TGFB2, MSX1, TGFA & TGAFB3 in the etiology of cleft lip and palate in the Philippines. Cleft Palate Craniofac J. 1997:34:1-6.

6. Ardinger et al. Association of genetic variation of the transforming growth factor – alpha gene with CL / CP. Am J Hum genet. 1989: 45: 348-353.

7. Aramany MA. A history of prosthetic management of cleft palate: pare to swerson. Cleft Palate J. 1971; 8: 415-430.

8. Bailey et al: Carbon monoxide effects on cleft lip development in mice. J Dent Res, 1988:67:194.

9. Bardach J, Cutting CB. Anatomy of the unilateral and bilateral cleft lip and nose. In Bardach J.Morris HL, Eds. Multidisciplinary management of cleft lip and palate. Philadelphia WB Saunders: 1990; 150-159.

10. Barry L Eppley et al. Management of alveolar cleft bone grafting – State of the art. Cleft Palate Croniofac J. 2000; 37; 229-233.

11. Bixler D. Genetics and clefting. Cleft Palate J: 1981: 18;10-18.

12. Bluestone CD, Beery QC, Cantekin EI, and Paradise JL: Eustachian tube ventilatory function in relation to cleft palate. Annals of Otology 84:333-338,1975.

13. Boustrad; Minimally invasive iliac cancellous bone graft harvesting. Plast Reconst Surg. 1997; 99; 1769-1761.

14. Boyne and Sands. Secondary bone grafting of residual alveolar and palatal clefts. J Oral Maxillofac Surg. 1972; 30; 87-92.

15. Braganza RA, Kearns DB, Button DM, Seid AB, and Pruzansky SM: Closure of the soft palate for persistent otorrhea after placement of pressure equalization tubes in cleft palate infants. Cleft Palate Craniofac. 28:305-307, 1991.

16. Brecht et al. Columellar elongation in the bilateral cleft lip and nose patient. J Dent Res 1995; 74; 257.

17. Bretherton. Attachment theory; retrospect and prospect. Monogr Soc Res Child Dev 1985; 50; 3-35.

18. Broder et al. Learning disability, school achivement, and grade retention among children with CL / CP, a two center study. Cleft Palate Craniofac J. 1998;35;127-131.

19. Broder HL et al. Self concept of early primary school age children with visible or invisible defects. Cleft Palate J. 26:114-117, 1989.

20. Broder HL, Smith FB, and Strauss RP: Effects of visible and invisible orofacial defects on self-perception and adjustment across development and gender. Cleft Palate Craniofac J.. 31:429-436, 1994.

21. Boone DR, and McFarlane SC: The voice and voice therapy, Englewood Cliffs (NJ): Prentice-Hall, 1994.

22. Broen PA, Doyle SS, and Bacon CK : The velopharyngeally inadequate child: Phonologic change with intervention. Cleft Palate Craniofac J. 30:500-507, 1993.

23. Bronsky. Morphogenesis of hypoxia induced cleft lip in CL/fr mice. J Craniofac Genet Dev Biol. 1986; 2; 113.

24. Burston, W.R.: The early orthodontic treatment of cleft palate conditions. Dent Pract (Bristol), 9:41, 1958.

25. Catharina Jacobsson. Effects of B6 on Beta – Aminoproprinonitrile induced palatal cleft formation in the rat. Cleft Palate Craniofac J. 1997:34:95-100.

26. Catherine L Marie et al. Are infants without orofacial clefts at risk for insecure mother–child attachments? Cleft Palate Cranifac J. 2000;31;257-266.

27. Christensen K. The 20th Century Darnish facial cleft population- epidemilogial and genetic – epidemiological studies. Cleft Palate Craniofac J. 1999; 36; 96-104.

28. Chung et al. Genetic epidemiology of cleft lip with or without palate in the population of Hawaii. Genet Epidemiol. 1987;4;415-423

29. Clarren et al: The fetal alcohol syndrome. N Engl J Med. 1978; 298; 1063-1067.

30. Clifford E: Psychological aspects of cleft lip and palate. In Bzoch KR (ed). Communicative disorders related to CL/P 2nd ed. Voston: Little Brown. 1979 37-51.

31. Cobley. Modification of the Koken nasal splint. Cleft Palate Craniofac J. 2000; 37; 125-126

32. Coccano, P.J.: Orthodontics in cleft palate children: a continuing process. Cleft Palate J., 6:495, 1970.

33. Cohen M Polley; Secondary (Intermediate) alveolar bone grafting. Cin Plast Surg. 1993; 4; 691-705

34. Cohen MM Jr. The child with multiple birth defects. New York: Raven Press; 1982.

35. Conway H. Effect of supplemental vitamin therapy on the limitation of incidence of cleft lip and CP in human; Plast Reconstr Surg. 1958; 28; 450-453.

36. Croen et al. Racial and ethnic variations in the prevalence of orofacial clefts in California, 1983–1992. Am J Med Genet. 1998; 79; 42-47.

37. Cutting et al. Presurgical columellar elongation and primary retrograde nasal reconstruction in one stage bilateral cleft lip and nose repair. Plast Reconstr Surg. 1998; 101; 630-639.

38. David J Reisbegg. Dental and prosthetic care for patients with cleft or craniofacial conditions. Cleft Palate Cranifac J. 2000; 37; 534-537
39. De Voss H: A Study of the factors relative to the incidence of cleft palate births from 1945 through 1949 in San Bernadio country. Speech Monographs. 19:303-308,1952
40. Desault, P.J., and Bichat, X.: Sur l'operaion du bec-de-lievre. In Oeuvres Chirurgicales ou Expose de la Doctrine et de la Plastique. Vol. 2. Paris, Megengnon, 1798.
41. Diego F Wyszynski et al: Use of U.S. birth certificate data to estimate the risk of maternal cigarratte smoking for oral clefting. Cleft Palate Craniofac J. 2002:39:188-192
42. Dostal et al. Further studies on protective effects of vitamins in cyclphospamide–induced CP. Int J Oral Maxillofac. Surg. 1990; 19; 308-311.
43. Drillien, C.M., Ingram, T.T.S., and Walkinson, E.M.: The causes and natural history of cleft lip and palate. Edinburgh, E. and S. Livingstone, 1966.
44. Eliason MJ: Cleft lip and palate developmental effects. Journal of Pediatric Nursing. 5:107-113, 1991.
45. Endriga MC, and Kapp-Simon KA: Psychological issues in craniofacial care: state of the art. Cleft Palate Craniofacial journal. 36: 3-33, 1999.
46. Erickson et al: Cigarrette smoking as an etiologic factor in cleft lip and palate. Am J Doster Gynecol. 1979; 135-138.
47. Fisk SB, Pearl RM, Schulman GI, and Wong H: Craniofacial anomalies among 4 through 7 year olds: psychological effects and surgical decisions. Annals of Plastic Surgery: 14:37-42, 1985.
48. Fogh-Andersen P: Inheritance of harelip and cleft palate, Copenhagen: Munksgaard, 1942.
49. Fogh-Andersen, P.: Inheritance of harelip and cleft palate. Copenjagen, Nyt Nordisk Forlag, Arnold Busck, 1942.
50. Frank et al. Teratogenicity of 3,3 dimethyl – 1 – phenyl triazone in the rat gross malformations including micrognathism. Teratology. 1989; 39; 53-61
51. Fraser, F.C.: The genetics of cleft lip and palate. Am J Hum Genet. 22:336, 1970.
52. Fraser, G.R., and Calnan, J.S.: Cleft lip and palate: seasonal incidence, birth weight, birth rank, sex, site, associated malformations and parental age. Arch Dis Child. 36:420, 1961.
53. Fujino, H., Tanaka, K., and Sanui, Y.: Genetic study of clet lips and cleft palates based on 2828 Japanese cases. Kyushu J. Med. Sci., 14:317, 1963.
54. Gary M Shaw et al. Infant TGF – alpha genotypes orofacial clefts and maternal periconceptional multi-vitamin use. Cleft Palate Craniofac J.1998; 35; 366 – 370.
55. Geoffrey H Sperber – Craniofacial Embryology. 1989,132-141.
56. Georgiade. N. G. Improved technique for one stage repair of bilateral cleft lip. Plast Reconstr Surg., 48:318, 1971.
57. Grabowski. Embryonic O_2 deficiency – a physilogical approch to analysis of teratological mechanism. Adv Teratol 4:125,1970.

58. Grayson et al. Presurgical nasoalveolar moulding in infant with cleft lip and palate. Cleft Palate Craniofac J. 1999, 36: 486-498.
59. Guntler Schultes et al. Comparison of periodontal disease in patients without cleft of palate and patients with unilateral clefts of lip palate and alveolus. Cleft Palate Craniofac J 1999; 39; 322-327.
60. Harkins, C.S.: Principles of cleft oalate prosthesis. Philadelphia, Temple University Press, 1960.
61. Harper D and Richman LC: Personality profiles of physically impaired adolescents. Journal of Clinical psychology 34:636-642, 1978.
62. Henningsson EG, and Isberg AM: Velopharyngeal movement pattern in patients alternating between oral and glottal articulation: a clinical and cineradiographical study. Cleft Palate J. 23:1-9, 1986.
63. Hicks et al: Maternal phenytion administration affects DNA and protein synthesis in enbryonic primary palates. Teratology. 1983, 28-389.
64. Ingalls, T.H., Taube, I.E., and Klinberg, M.A.: Cleft lip and cleft palate: epidemiologic considerations: Plast, Reconstr. Surg., 34:1, 1964.
65. Ivy, R. H.: The influence of race on the incidence of certain congenital anomalies notably cleft lip and cleft palate. Plast, Reconstr. Surg., 30:581, 1962.
66. Jaksi D.N. Mesiodistal size of deciduous teeth in subject with unilateral cleft lip and palate. Orthod craniofacRes 2002; Feb, 5; 17-21.
67. Jennifer L Graw. A local perspective as the initial management of children with cleft lip and palate by primary care physicians. Cleft Palate Craniofac J. 2002, 39: 535-541.
68. Jonathan A Britto. Toward pathogenesis of apert cleft palate; FGF, FGFR, and TGFB genes are differentially expressed in sequential stages of human palatal shelf fusion. Cleft Palate Craniofac J. 2002; 39; 332-340.
69. Joseph G Mc.Carthy. Cleft lip and palate and Craniofacial Anomalies. 1990:Vol 4.
70. Kaare Christensen et al. Facial clefting and psychiatric disease; a follow up of the Danish 1936-1987 facial cleft cohort. Cleft Palate Craniofac J. 2002:39:392-397.
71. Kaehn DP: New therapy for treating hypernasal speech using continuous positive airway pressure (CPAP). Plastic and Reconstructive Surgery 88:959-966, 1991.
72. Kang et al. Intermediate hyper homocysteinemia resulting from compound heterozygosity of methylene tetrahydrofolate reductase mutations. Am J Hum Genet. 1991; 48; 546-551.
73. Kapp-Simon KA, Simon DJ, and Kristovich S: Self-perception, social skills, adjustment and inhibition in young adolescents with craniofacial anomalies. Clefts Palate Journal. 29:340-35, 1992.
74. Kapp–Simon. Self-concept of primary school age children with cleft lip, cleft palate or both cleft palates. Cleft Palate Craniofac J. 1986; 23; 24-27.
75. Kapp–Simon. Observed social interaction patterns in adolescents with and without craniofacial conditions. Cleft Palate Craniofac J. 1997; 34 ; 380-384.

76. Karin Kallen Maternal smoking and orofacial clefts. Cleft Palate Craniofac J 1997: 34:11-16

77. Krueckeberg SM and Kapp-Simon KA: Effect of parental factors on social skills of preschool children with craniofacial anomalies. Cleft palate Craniofac J. 30:490-496, 1993.

78. Latham, R.A., Kusy, R.P., and Georgiade, N.G.: An extraorally activated expansion appliance for cleft palate infants. Cleft Palate J., 13:253, 1976.

79. Lauder et al: Serotorin and morphogenesis .I. sites of serotonin uptake and binding protein immuno reactivity in the mid-gestation mouse embryo. Development, 102'709, 1988

80. LaVelle WE and Van Denmark: Construction of a maxillary orthopedic prosthesis for simultaneous maxillary expansion and obturation. Journal of Prosthetic Dentistry 35:665-670, 1976

81. Leslie Turner et al. The Effects of lactation education and a prosthetic obturator appliance on feeding in infants with CL / CP. Cleft Palate Craniofac J. 2002, 38; 519-524

82. Long et al: The effect of cuspid positioning in the cleft at the time of secondary bone grafting on eventual success. Cleft Palate Craniofac J. 1996; 33; 225-230.

83. Lowry and Trimble. Incidence rates for CL and P in British Columbia 1952-1971 for North American Indian Japanese, Chinese and Total populations; Secular trends over 20 years. Teratology 1977; 16; 277-284.

84. Lutz K. and Moore F: A study of factors in the occu\rrence of cleft palate. Journal of speech and Hearing Disorders 20:271-276, 1955.

85. Mackler: Studies of the developmental anomalies in rats. III. Effects of inhibition systems on embryonic development Teratology.1975, 12; 291.

86. Marazita ML.Genome scan for loci involved in CL with or without CP in Chinese multiplex families. Am J Hum Genet 2002 Aug. 71; 349-64.

87. Matsuo K et al. Preoperative non-surgical over–correction of cleft lip nasal deformity. Br J Plast Surg. 1991; 44; 5-11.

88. Maull et al. Long-term effects of nasoalveolar moulding presented at the annual meeting of the American Cleft Palate Craniofacial Association: New Orleans 1997.

89. McNeil, C.K.: Congenital oral deformities. Br. Dent. J. 101:191, 1956.

90. McNeil, C.K.: Oral and Facial Deformity, London, Pitman, 1954.

91. Mc Williams BJ: Cleft palate. In shames G, and Wing E (Eds) Human communication disorders, Columbus (OH): CE Merrill, 1982.

92. McWilliams BJ, and Philips BJ; Audio seminars in speech pathology velopharyngeal incompetence. Toronoto: BC Decker, 1979:1989:1990.

93. McWilliams BJ: Social and psychological problems associated with cleft palate. Clinics in Plastic Surgery: Symposium on social and psychological consideration in Plastic Surgery 9:317-326, 1982.

94. McWilliams, B. J., Morris, H.L., and Shelton, R.L. (Eds.): Cleft Palate Speech. Philadelphia, B.C. Decker; St. Louis, C.V. Mosby, 1984.

95. Michael C. Rapid Palatal expansion in adults with and without surgery. Angle Orthodontist 1987; 3; 245-263.

96. Mikihiko Kogo et al. Breast-feeding for cleft lip and palate patients using Hotz–type plate. Cleft Palate Craniofac J. 1997, 34; 351-353.

97. Millard and Latharn. Improved primary surgical and dental treatment of clefts. Plast Recort Surg. 1990,86; 856.

98. Miller TJ. CP formation a role for pyridoxine in the closure of the secondary palate in mice. Teratology 1972; 6; 351-356.

99. Millicovsky et al. Hyperoxia and hypoxia in pregnancy simple experimental manipulation alters the incidence of cleft lip and palate in CL/Fr mice. Proc Natl Acad. Sci; USA; 1981; 78; 5722.

100. Moore IJ, Moore GF, and Yonkers AJ: Otitis media in the cleft palate patient. Ear, Nose and Throat, Journal. 65:15-23, 1986.

101. Moore RB: Orthodontic management of the patient with cleft lip and palate. Ear, Nose and Throat Journal. 65:46-58, 1986.

102. Morley ME: Cleft palate and speech 7th Ed, Baltimore: Williams and Wilkins 1970.

103. Murray JC. Face facts genes, environment and clefts. Am J Hum Genet. 1995, 57'227-232.

104. Natalie J Prescott et al. Folate and the face: Evaluating the guidence for the influence of folate genes on craniofacial development. Cleft Palate Craniofac J. 2002, 39; 327-331.

105. Neel, J.V.: A study of major congenital defects in Japanese infants. Am. J. Hum. Genet. 10:398, 1958.

106. Nunn DR, Derkay CS, Darrow DH, Magee W, and Strasnick B: The effect of very early cleft palate closure on the need for ventilation tubes in the first year of life. Laryngoscope. 105:9050908, 1995.

107. Ortiz-Posadas et al: A new approach to classify cleft lip and palate. Cleft Palate Craniofac J. 2001; 38; 545-550.

108. Pedro E Santigo. Reduced need for alveolar bone grafting by presurgical orthopedics and primary gigivoplasty. Cleft Palate Craniofac J. 1998; 35; 77-80.

109. Peer et al. Effect of vitamins on human teratology. Plast Reconstr Surg. 1964:34:358-362.

110. Peterson-Falzone SJ: Compensatory articulations in cleft palate speakers: relative incidence by type. Proceedings of the international Congress on cleft palate and related craniofacial anomalies. Jerusalem, Israel, 1989.

111. Peterson – Falzone. Cleft Palate Speech .2001 3rd Edison.

112. Peterson – Falzone SJ: Resonance disorders in structural defects. In Lass NJ, McReynolds LV, Northern JL, and Yolder DE (eds): Speech language and hearing, volume II: Pathologies of speech and language Philadelphia: WB Saunders 1982.

113. Peterson et al. Contemporary Oral Maxillofacial Surgery 2nd edi. 1997, 663-667.

114. Pope AW, and Ward J: Factors associated with peer social competence in preadolescents with craniofacial anomalies. Journal of Pediatric Psychology 22:455-470, 1997.

115. Pope AW; Points of risk and opportunity for parents of children with craniofacial conditions. Cleft Palate Craniofac J. 36:36-39, 1999.

116. Pruzansky, S., and Aduss, H.: Prevalence of arch collapse and malocclusion in complete unilaterlal cleft lip and palate. Trans. Eur. Orthod. Soc., 1:16. 1967.

117. Ralph E Mc Donald et al: Dentisty for the Child and Adolescent 1996 5th Edition.

118. Ralph Millard Jr. Cleft craft. The evaluation of its surgery. I the unilateral deformity 1st edition 57-67: 1976.

119. Ren et al. Velopharyngeal incompetence and persistant hypernansality after adenoidectomy in children wihtout palatal defects. Cleft Palate Craniofac J. 1995; 32; 476-482.

120. Richman LC. Facial and speech relationship to behaviour of children with clefts across three age levels. Cleft Palate Craniofac J. 1997:34:390-395.

121. Richman LC, and Millard TI: Cleft lip and palate longitudinal behaviour and relationship of cleft conditions to behaviour and achievement. Journal of Pediatric Psychology 22:487-494, 1997.

122. Richman LC, Holmes CS, and Eliason Mj, and Lindgren SC: Reading disability in children with clefts. Cleft Palate J. 25:21-25, 1988.

123. Rintala et al: On the pathogenesis of cleft palate in the Pierre Robin syndrome Scand. J Plast Reconstrsurg. 1984; 18; 237-240.

124. Riski JE: Functional velopharyngeal incompetence: diagnosis and management. In winitz H (ed): treating articulations disorders for clinicians by clinicians. Baltimore, University, Park Press, 1984.

125. Rojer K.Hall. Pediatric Orofacial Medicine and Pathology. Chpman and Hall Publications. 1994.

126. Ronald P Strauss: Beyond easy answers: prenatal diagnosis and counselling during pregnancy. Cleft Palate Craniofac J. 2002:39; 164-169.

127. Rubin and Wilkinson – Peer rejection and social isolation in childhood: a conceptually inspired research agenda for children with croniofacial handicaps. In Eder RA ed. Craniofacial Anomalies; Psychological perspectives. New York Springer Verlag: 1995:158-176.

128. Ruscello DM, Shuster LI, and Sandwisch A: Modification of context specific nasal emission. Journal of Speech and Hearing Research 34:27-32, 1991.

129. Rynnel. Dagoo B, Lindberg K, Bagger. Sjoback D and Larson O: Middle ear disease in cleft palate children at three years of age. International Journal of Pediatric Otorhinolaryngology. 23:201-209, 1992.

130. Sadove et al: An evaluation of clavical and illiac donor sites in alveolar cleft grafting: a surgeon's view–point plast reconstr Surg. 1982: 70: 297-307.

131. Samir E. Bishara et al: Dentofacial findings in two individual with unoperated bilateral cleft lip. AJO-DO. 1985 Jul 22-30.

132. Samuel Stal. Classic and occult Submucous cleft palates: A histopathalogic analysis. Cleft Palate Croniojac J. 1998:35:351-358.

133. Santiago et al: Reduced need for alveolar bone grafting by presurgical orthodontics and primary gingivoperisteo plasty. Cleft Palate Craniofac J. 1998; 35; 77-80.

134. Shprintzen R, McCall GM, and Skolnick J: A new therapeutic technique for the treatment of velopharyngeal incompetence. Journal of Speech and Hearing Disorders. 40; 69-83, 1975.

135. Shwa et al. Ethical and Scientific decision-making in distraction osteogenesis. Cleft Palate Craniofac J. 2002; 39; 641-646.

136. Siva Raju S. In research of a smile, Study of children born with cleft lip and palate in India. 2000; 7; 32.

137. Skoog T.The use of periosteal flaps in the repair of cleft of the primary palate. Cleft Palate J. 1965;2;332.

138. Smith TL, DiRuggiero DC, and Jones KR: Recovery of Eustachian tube function and hearing outcomes in patients with cleft palate. Otolaryngology – Head and Neck surgery, 111:423-429, 1994.

139. Speltz et al: Psychological functioning of children with craniofacial anomalies and their mothers -a follow up from late infancy to school entry. Cleft Palate Craniofac J. 1993; 30 482-489.

140. Spriestersbach, D.C., Lierle, D.M., Moll, K.L., and Prather. W. F.: Hearing loss in children with cleft palates. Plast Reconstr Surg. 30:336, 1962.

141. Stoll et al. Associated malformations in cases with oral clefts. Cleft Palate Craniofac J. 2000:37:43-48.

142. Stool SE, and Winn R: Pneumatization of the temporal bone in children with cleft palate: Cleft Palate Journal. 6:154-159, 1969.

143. Stool SE, Research revisited. Cleft Palate Journal 26:344-345, 1989.

144. Strauss RP, and Broder HL, Directions and issues in psychosocial research and methods as applied to cleft lip and palate and craniofacial anomalies. Clefts Palate Craniofac J. 28:150-156, 1991.

145. Sulik et al. Phenytoin induced CL / CP in A/J mices a scanning and transmission electron microsopic study. Anat Rec. 1979 195:243.

146. Tatsuo N et al. Augmentation of the nostril splint for retaining the corrected contour of the cleft lip nose. Plast Reconstr Surg. 1990:85:182-186.

147. Timorhty A Turvey et al. Facial clefts and cranio synostosis, principles and management. 1996 1st edition 135-137.

148. Tobiasen JM: Psychosocical adjustment to cleft lip and palate. In Bardach J and Morris HL (eds): Multidisciplinary management of cleft lip and palate Philadelphia: WB Saunders, 1990: 820-825.

149. Tobiasen JM, and Hiebert JM: Clefting and psychological adjustment clinics in palate surgery. Advances in management of cleft Lip and palate 20:623-631, 1993.

150. Tolarova M: A study of the incidence sex-ratio, laterality, and clinical severity in 3,660 probands with facial clefts in Czechoslovakia, Acta Chirurgiae Platicae 19:77-87, 1987

151. Tolarova M: Periconceptional supplementation with vitamins and folic acid to prevent recurrence of cleft lip, Lancet 2:217, 1982

152. Trost-Cardamone JE: Speech anatomy, physiology and pathology. In Kernahan DA, and Rosenstein SW (eds) Cleft lip and palate a system of management, Baltimore: Williams, and Wilkins, 1990.

153. Trost-Cardamone JE: The development of speech assessing cleft palate misarticulations. In Kernahan DA, and Rosenstein SW (eds); Cleft lip and palate: a system of management Baltimore: Williams and Wilkins, 1990.

154. Trost-Cardamone JE: Diagnosis and management of speakers with craniofacial anomalies. Short course presented at the American Speech Language-Hearing Association Annual Covention. Orlando (FL) 1995.

155. Trost JE; Articulatory additions to the classical descriptions of the speech of persons with cleft palate. Cleft Palate J. 18:193-203, 1981.

156. Trost JE; Articulatory additions to the classical description of the speech of person with cleft palate. Cleft Palate J. 18:193-203. 1981.

157. Tyan ML: Difference in the reported frequencies of cleft lip plus cleft lip and palate in Asian born in Hawaii and the continental United States. Proceedings of the Society for Experimental Biology and Medicine. 171:41-45, 1982.

158. Van Demark DR. and Hardin M: Effectiveness of intensive articulation therapy for children with cleft palate. Cleft Palate J. 23:215-224, 1986.

159. Vanderas AP: Incidence of cleft lip, cleft palate, and cleft lip and palate among races- a review. Cleft Palate J. 24:216-225, 1987

160. Vargervik K; Orthodontic treatment of children with cleft lip and palate. In Barach J, and Shprintzen RJ (eds): Cleft palate speech management St.Louis; Mosby, 1995, 295-304.

161. Volker Bienengrber et al; Application of thiamine in preventing malformations, specifically cleft alveolus and palate during the intrauterine development of rats. Cleft Palate Craniofac J. 1997:34:318-324.

162. Werler et al: Maternal alcohol use in relation to selected birth defects. Am J Epidemiol. 1991: 134:691-698.

163. Wilson, M.E.: A ten-year survey of cleft lip and cleft palate in the South West region. Br. J.Plast. Surg., 25:224, 1972.

164. Witzel MA, Tobe J and Salyer K: The use of nasopharyngoscopy biofeedback therapy in the correction of inconsistent velopharyngeal closure. International Journal of Pediatric Otorhinolaryngology. 15:137-142, 1988.

165. Wolfe and Berkowitz: The use of cranial bone grafts in the closure of alveolar and palatal clefts. Plast reconstr surg. 1983: 72:659-666.

166. Wong et al; Non syndromic orofacial clefts: association with maternal hyperhomocystinemia. Teratology. 1999:60:253-257.

167. Wood et al; Gingivoperiosteoplasty and midfacial growth. Cleft Palate Craniofac J. 1997: 34:17-20.

168. Woolf, C.M. Woolf, R.M., and Broadbent, T.R.: Genetic and nongenetic variables related to cleft lip and palate. Plast Reconstr Surg. 232:65, 1963.

169. Woolf, C.M.: Paternal age effect for cleft lip and palate. Am J Hum Genet, 15:389, 1963.

170. Wyszinski et al. Genetics of nonsyndromic oral clefts revisited. Cleft Palate Craniofac J. 1996:33:406-417.
171. Yi NN. Epidermiology of cleft lip and palate in Singapore a 10-year hospital based study. Ann Acad Med Singapore. 1999:28:655-659.
172. Zhuman Bian. Caries experience and oral health behaviour in Chinese children with cleft lip and or palate. Am Acad Pediatr dent. 2001, 23:431-434.

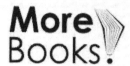
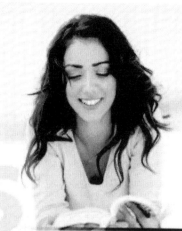
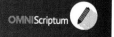

Printed in Great Britain
by Amazon

75897887R00079